*Effect of IL-10 and anti-TGF-beta
antibodies on the morphology of
bone marrow stroma cultures
from
Interleukin-10
by
Jan E. DeVries and
René de Waal Malefyt
© RG Landes Co. 1995*

MOLECULAR BIOLOGY INTELLIGENCE UNIT

CALRETICULIN

Marek Michalak, Ph.D.

MRC Group in Molecular Biology of Membranes
Department of Biochemistry
University of Alberta
Edmonton, Alberta, Canada

CHAPMAN & HALL
ITP An International Thomson Publishing Company

New York • Albany • Bonn • Boston • Cincinnati • Detroit • London • Madrid • Melbourne •
Mexico City • Pacific Grove • Paris • San Francisco • Singapore • Tokyo • Toronto • Washington

R.G. LANDES COMPANY
AUSTIN

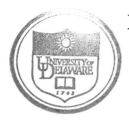

MOLECULAR BIOLOGY INTELLIGENCE UNIT

CALRETICULIN

R.G. LANDES COMPANY
Austin, Texas, U.S.A.

U.S. and Canada Copyright © 1996 R.G. Landes Company and Chapman & Hall
International Copyright © 1996 Springer-Verlag, Heidelberg, Germany

Please address all inquiries to the Publishers:
R.G. Landes Company, 909 Pine Street, Georgetown, Texas, U.S.A. 78626
Phone: 512/ 863 7762; FAX: 512/ 863 0081

Chapman & Hall, 115 Fifth Avenue, New York, New York, U.S.A. 10003

Springer-Verlag GmbH & Co. KG, Tiergartenstrasse 17, D-69121 Heidelberg, Germany

U.S. and Canada ISBN 0-412-10101-7
International ISBN 3-540-60429-4

While the authors, editors and publisher believe that drug selection and dosage and the specifications and usage of equipment and devices, as set forth in this book, are in accord with current recommendations and practice at the time of publication, they make no warranty, expressed or implied, with respect to material described in this book. In view of the ongoing research, equipment development, changes in governmental regulations and the rapid accumulation of information relating to the biomedical sciences, the reader is urged to carefully review and evaluate the information provided herein.

Library of Congress Cataloging-in-Publication Data

Calreticulin/ [edited by] Marek Michalak
    p. cm. — (Molecular biology intelligence unit)
  Includes bibliographical references and index.
  ISBN 0-412-10101-7 (alk. paper)
  1. Calreticulin. I. Michalak, Marek. II. Series.
QP552.C29C35 1995   95-38421
574.19'245--dc20   CIP

PUBLISHER'S NOTE

R.G. Landes Company publishes five book series: *Medical Intelligence Unit, Molecular Biology Intelligence Unit, Neuroscience Intelligence Unit, Tissue Engineering Intelligence Unit* and *Biotechnology Intelligence Unit.* The authors of our books are acknowledged leaders in their fields and the topics are unique. Almost without exception, no other similar books exist on these topics.

Our goal is to publish books in important and rapidly changing areas of medicine for sophisticated researchers and clinicians. To achieve this goal, we have accelerated our publishing program to conform to the fast pace in which information grows in biomedical science. Most of our books are published within 90 to 120 days of receipt of the manuscript. We would like to thank our readers for their continuing interest and welcome any comments or suggestions they may have for future books.

Deborah Muir Molsberry
Publications Director
R.G. Landes Company

Acknowledgments

I would like to thank my wife and my daughter for their patience and understanding. Many thanks to M. Opas for his friendship and continuing contribution to our work. I am grateful to the past and present members of our laboratory C. Andrin, S. Baksh, K. Burns, J. Busaan, M. Dabrowska, K. Famulskiu, L. Fliegel, S. Fu, J. Hance, N. Mesaeli, R. Milner, P. Nash, C. Shemanko, and M. Waser for many helpful discussions and for their contribution to various aspects of calreticulin research carried out in our laboratory. Many thanks to M. Waser for superb graphic designs and to R.E. Milner for help in editing and critical reading of the manuscripts. Research in our laboratory is supported by the MRC Group in Molecular Biology of Membranes, the Heart and the Stroke Foundation of Alberta, the Muscular Dystrophy Association of Canada and the Alberta Heritage Foundation for Medical Research.

CONTENTS

EDITOR

Marek Michalak, Ph.D.
MRC Group in Molecular Biology of Membranes
Department of Biochemistry
University of Alberta
Edmonton, Alberta, Canada
Chapters 1, 2

CONTRIBUTORS

Christi Andrin
MRC Group in Molecular Biology
   of Membranes
Department of Biochemistry
University of Alberta
Edmonton, Alberta, Canada
Chapter 1

Eric A. Atkinson, M.Sc.
Department of Biochemistry
University of Alberta
Edmonton, Alberta, Canada
Chapter 9

Chintamani D. Atreya, Ph.D.
Laboratory of Molecular
   Pharmacology
Center for Biologics Evaluation
   and Research
Food and Drug Administration
Bethesda, Maryland, USA
Chapter 7

Shairaz Baksh, Ph.D.
MRC Group in Molecular Biology
   of Membranes
Department of Pediatrics
University of Alberta
Edmonton, Alberta, Canada
Chapter 2

Claude Benedict, M.D.
Department of Medicine
University of Texas
Health Sciences Center at Houston
Houston, Texas, USA
Chapter 10

John J.M. Bergeron, D.Phil.
Department of Anatomy and
   Cell Biology
McGill University
Montreal, Quebec, Canada
Chapter 4

R. Chris Bleackley, Ph.D.
Department of Biochemistry
University of Alberta
Edmondton, Alberta, Canada
Chapter 9

Johan Broekmann, Ph.D.
Department of Medicine
Cornell University Medical Center
New York, New York, USA
Chapter 10

CONTRIBUTORS

J. Donald Capra, M.D.
Department of Microbiology
University of Texas Southwestern
  Medical Center
Dallas, Texas, USA
Chapter 8

Shih-Tsung Cheng, M.D.
Department of Dermatology
University of Texas Southwestern
  Medical Center
Dallas, Texas, USA
Chapter 8

Victor B. Hatcher, Ph.D.
Departments of Biochemistry
  and Medicine
Albert Einstein College of Medicine
Montefiore Medical Center
Bronx, New York, USA
Chapter 12

Richard Hemming, Ph.D.
Genetics Group, Biotechnology
  Research Institute
National Research Council
  of Canada
Department of Anatomy and Cell
  Biology
McGill University
Montreal, Quebec, Canada
Chapter 4

Deborah C. Jaworski, Ph.D.
Department of Molecular Biology
  and Biochemistry
University of California, Irvine
Irvine, California, USA
Chapter 11

Karl-Heinz Krause, M.D.
Division of Infectious Diseases
University Hospital
Geneva, Switzerland
Chapter 5

Keisuke Kuwabara, M.D.
Department of Neuroradiology
Osaka University Medical Center
Osaka, Japan
Chapter 10

Charles A. Lawson, M.D.
Department of Physiology
  and Cellular Biophysics
College of Physicians and Surgeons
  of Columbia University
New York, New York, USA
Chapter 10

Tsu-San Lieu, Ph.D.
Department of Dermatology
University of Texas Southwestern
  Medical Center
Dallas, Texas, USA
Chapter 8

Tadeusz Malinski, Ph.D.
Department of Biology
University of Oakland
Oakland, Michigan, USA
Chapter 10

Aaron J. Marcus, M.D.
Department of Medicine
Cornell University Medical Center
New York, New York, USA
Chapter 10

CONTRIBUTORS

Nasrin Mesaeli, Ph.D.
MRC Group in Molecular
    Biology of Membranes
Department of Biochemistry
University of Alberta
Edmonton, Alberta, Canada
Chapter 6

Hira L. Nakhasi, Ph.D.
Laboratory of Molecular
    Pharmacology
Division of Hematologic Products
Center for Biologics Evaluation
    and Research
Food and Drug Administration
Bethesda, Maryland, USA
Chapter 7

Glen R. Needham, Ph.D.
Department of Entomology
The Ohio State University
Columbus, Ohio, USA
Chapter 11

Tho Q. Nguyen, M.D.
Department of Dermatology
University of Texas Southwestern
    Medical Center
Dallas, Texas, USA
Chapter 8

Michal Opas, Ph.D.
Department of Anatomy
    and Cell Biology
University of Toronto
Toronto, Ontario, Canada
Chapter 3

Wei-Jia Ou, Ph.D.
Genetics Group, Biotechnology
    Research Institute
National Research Council of Canada
Department of Anatomy
    and Cell Biology
McGill University
Montreal, Quebec, Canada
Chapter 4

Frank Parlati
Genetics Group, Biotechnology
    Research Institute
National Research Council of Canada
Department of Biology
McGill University
Montreal, Quebec, Canada
Chapter 4

Michael J. Pinkoski, M.Sc.
Department of Biochemistry
University of Alberta
Edmonton, Alberta, Canada
Chapter 9

David J. Pinsky, M.D.
Department of Medicine
College of Physicians and Surgeons
    of Columbia University
New York, New York, USA
Chapter 10

Gregory P. Pogue, Ph.D.
Laboratory of Molecular Pharmacology
Center for Biologics Evaluation
    and Research
Food and Drug Administration
Bethesda, Maryland, USA
Chapter 7

CONTRIBUTORS

Jane Ryan, Ph.D.
Department of Physiology
  and Cellular Biophysics
College of Physicians and Surgeons
  of Columbia University
New York, New York, USA
Chapter 10

Christina Samathanam, Ph.D.
Department of Biochemistry
Albert Einstein College
  of Medicine
Bronx, New York, USA
Chapter 12

Ann Marie Schmidt, M.D.
Department of Physiology
  and Cellular Biophysics
College of Physicians and Surgeons
  of Columbia University
New York, New York, USA
Chapter 10

Nishi K. Singh, Ph.D.
Laboratory of Molecular
  Pharmacology
Center for Biologics Evaluation
  and Research
Food and Drug Administration
Bethesda, Maryland, USA
Chapter 7

Richard D. Sontheimer, M.D.
Department of Dermatology
University of Texas Southwestern
  Medical Center
Dallas, Texas, USA
Chapter 8

David M. Stern, M.D.
Department of Physiology
  and Cellular Biophysics
College of Physicians and Surgeons
  of Columbia University
New York, New York, USA
Chapter 10

David Y. Thomas, Ph.D.
Genetics Group, Biotechnology
  Research Institute
National Research Council of Canada
Department of Anatomy
  and Cell Biology
Department of Biology
McGill University
Montreal, Quebec, Canada
Chapter 4

PREFACE

In the early 70s, while studying calcium binding proteins of muscle sarcoplasmic reticulum, MacLennan's group at the University of Toronto identified and characterized several soluble calcium binding proteins. One of these proteins bound calcium with a relatively high affinity and was, therefore, named the high affinity calcium binding protein. About 20 years later we realized that this protein is only a minor component of muscle sarcoplasmic reticulum, but is a major calcium binding protein of non-muscle endoplasmic reticulum. The next major breakthrough in calreticulin's research was the molecular cloning of the protein in 1989 and the realization that the protein has independently been "rediscovered" under a variety of different names by a number of investigators studying diverse areas of biology. The name calreticulin was universally adopted and it rapidly became clear that calreticulin may play an important role in virtually every aspect of cell biology.

Reading this book, many investigators may be be surprised to discover the significance of calreticulin in their area of research. From calcium binding/storage to cytotoxic T-cell function, from antithrombotic activity to tick physiology, from control of gene expression to nuclear import, from autoimmunity to viral replication encompass just a few amazing features of calreticulin. How can calreticulin, an endoplasmic reticulum protein, be involved in so many cellular processes? The book raises many more intriguing questions and gives a unique opportunity to realize the significance of calreticulin.

CHAPTER 1

A CURRENT HISTORY OF CALRETICULIN

Marek Michalak and Christi Andrin

INTRODUCTION

Ca^{2+} plays a vital role as a second messenger in virtually all eukaryotic cells. Changes in the intracellular concentration of Ca^{2+}, triggered by hormonal or electrical signals, elicit responses as diverse as contraction, cellular proliferation, secretion, metabolism adjustment, apoptosis, autoimmunity and changes in gene expression. Considering the diversity of the biological processes regulated by Ca^{2+}, it is not surprising that many investigators have devoted their research entirely to Ca^{2+}-binding proteins.

HACBP

In the early 1970s MacLennan's group isolated and characterized two Ca^{2+} binding proteins in muscle sarcoplasmic reticulum. One, a major, high-capacity Ca^{2+} binding (sequestering) protein of the muscle sarcoplasmic reticulum, was named calsequestrin.[1] The other bound Ca^{2+} not only with high capacity but also with a relatively high affinity[2] and, accordingly, was named the high affinity Ca^{2+} binding protein (HACBP).[2] At the time, in comparison with calsequestrin, the HACBP did not receive much attention. Since it bound Ca^{2+} with a relatively high affinity (μM) but was localized in the lumen of the sarcoplasmic reticulum (an environment then believed to contain millimolar concentrations of Ca^{2+}), its high affinity Ca^{2+} binding behaviour was considered unlikely to be of any physiological relevance.

Late in 1978 I (MM) joined David MacLennan's group as a postdoctoral fellow. He suggested I work with the HACBP and attempt to sort out its function. It proved difficult to work with. The purification procedure was lengthy and yielded relatively small amounts of material. Production of antibodies and immunoprecipitation were also very difficult. Further, we discovered that the protein was only a minor component of the sarcoplasmic reticulum.[3] When I completed my research training in David's laboratory there was not much interest in the HACBP.

CALREGULIN

In 1985 David Waisman reported the isolation and characterization of a new Ca^{2+} binding protein from bovine liver.[4] He named the protein calregulin, in anticipation that it might play some Ca^{2+}-dependent, regulatory role. Waisman's group carried out extensive physicochemical characterization of this protein, followed by quantitative radio-immunological analysis of its tissue distribution.[5,6] Waisman's group purified the protein from different sources and reported its N-terminal amino acid sequence.[7] Since immunocytochemical studies indicated that calregulin might be an endoplasmic reticulum protein,[5] the investigators became concerned that calregulin might be identical to calsequestrin, the major Ca^{2+} binding protein of muscle sarcoplasmic reticulum. However, thorough biochemical analysis revealed that calregulin was quite different from calsequestrin. Despite this, the investigators were unable to identify a physiological role for the protein, and at this stage, no comparison was made between calregulin and the HACBP.

CRP55

While studying Ca^{2+} binding proteins of the endoplasmic reticulum, Koch's group,[8] in Cambridge, identified a set of proteins which they referred to as reticuloplasmin. One of these proteins had a relatively high capacity for Ca^{2+} binding and was named CRP55 (calcium binding reticuloplasmin of molecular weight 55,000). Although biochemical and biophysical information concerning CRP55 was limited, Koch proposed that it might be analogous to muscle calsequestrin. Again, no comparison was made between this protein and the HACBP. In 1989 Smith and Koch[9] published the amino acid sequence of CRP55, and, at the same time, we published the amino acid sequence of the HACBP.[10] Only then was it realized that these proteins are identical.

CALRETICULIN

In 1987 our laboratory moved to the University of Alberta. Larry Fliegel had just completed molecular cloning of skeletal muscle calsequestrin in David MacLennan's laboratory and joined me in Edmonton. At this stage we decided to "play" with the HACBP again. There were, after all, some obvious questions to be answered. Is the HACBP a muscle or a nonmuscle protein? Is it similar to calsequestrin? Is it a functional/structural analog of calsequestrin? What is its function?

Larry decided to clone the protein, since we thought that this might provide some clues as to its physiological role. Early in 1988, a short cDNA clone was isolated from a rabbit skeletal muscle lambda gt11 expression library. Examination of the partial cDNA clone revealed that the C-terminus of the protein contained a large number of negatively charged amino acids and terminated with the endoplasmic reticulum retention signal, KDEL.[11] This was an exciting observation, since at this time, Pelham[12] had only just established that the C-terminal amino acid sequence KDEL is responsible for the retention of proteins resident in the endoplasmic reticulum. These observations enabled us to suggest that the HACBP must be resident in the lumen of the endoplasmic reticulum. This was confirmed by Michal Opas (University of Toronto) who was investigating the intracellular distribution of the HACBP, in both muscle and non-muscle systems (Chapter 3). This information led us to feel that the name HACBP was rather misleading. We proposed that the protein be re-named reticulin, to indicate its localization to the endoplasmic and sarcoplasmic reticulum.[13] Our molecular cloning of "reticulin" was completed by the end of 1988.[10] In addition, we performed N-terminal amino acid sequence analysis of the protein purified from uterine muscle and showed that this amino acid sequence was identical to that reported for calregulin. Simultaneously cDNA encoding mouse CRP55 was isolated in Cambridge by Koch's group. The cDNA confirmed the identity of CRP55 with both the HACBP and calregulin.[9] In 1990, McCauliffe et al[14] and Murthy et al[15] reported isolation of cDNA encoding human and rat forms of the protein, respectively.

By 1990 it was clear that, although the HACBP is only a minor component of muscle cells, it is a major Ca^{2+} binding protein in non-muscle endoplasmic reticulum. After consultation between David Waisman's group in Calgary, Gordon Koch's group in

Cambridge and our group in Edmonton the name calreticulin was adopted for the protein, to reflect its Ca^{2+} binding properties and its localization to the endo(sarco)plasmic reticulum. This name is now widely accepted.

RECENT OBSERVATIONS
AND UNANSWERED QUESTIONS

Some twenty years after its discovery, the function of calreticulin is still not known. Nevertheless, over the last few years many fascinating, somewhat intriguing observations have been made concerning this protein. For example, despite its endoplasmic reticulum retention signal, KDEL, it has been found in other parts of the cell. It has also been found to have a high degree of homology with several other proteins, suggesting that there may be an entire family of "calreticulin-like" proteins. Finally, it has been implicated in several quite diverse cellular functions.

Calreticulin has an N-terminal amino acid signal sequence and a C-terminal KDEL endoplasmic reticulum retention signal. It is, therefore, not surprising that calreticulin is localized to the lumen of the endoplasmic reticulum. However, experimental observations have revealed that it is also found in the nuclear envelope,[16] in cytoplasmic granules,[17] at the cell surface[18,19] and it may even be secreted into the blood stream.[20] To further complicate the story, calreticulin is found in tick saliva (Chapter 11),[21] sperm acrosomes,[22] and higher plants.[23,24] A calreticulin "family member" may also be the Joro spider toxin binding protein.[25] These observations pose several, as yet unanswered, questions. For example, does calreticulin have distinct functions in these distinct locations? Is calreticulin's ability to bind Ca^{2+} the key to its function in these different locations? How does calreticulin circumvent retention in the endoplasmic reticulum via its KDEL retention signal?

While calreticulin was originally identified as a Ca^{2+} binding protein, and plausible arguments suggest that it could have a role in Ca^{2+} homeostasis in the endoplasmic reticulum (Chapter 5), it has also, more recently, been shown to bind zinc[5] and iron.[26] This makes it possible that calreticulin could play a role in the control of other ion concentrations in different areas of the cell. Alternatively, some evidence indicates that calreticulin may act as a chaperone (Chapter 4).[27,28] This observation is interesting because another protein of the endoplasmic reticulum, calnexin, which shows some homology to calreticulin, also has chaperone activity (Chapter 4). Calreticulin has also been shown to have anti-thrombotic activity[29] (Chapter 10), but, at the same time, has marked homology with the *Aplysia* "memory molecule".[30]

The recent localization of calreticulin to the lytic granules of cytolytic T cells presents a whole new set of questions (Chapter 9).[17] Its function here is also unknown, but it may interact with perforin. Perforin, a protein centrally involved in the lysis of target cells, is activated by a precisely-timed exposure to Ca^{2+}. It is, therefore, not surprising that calreticulin, a Ca^{2+} binding protein, may be associated with this protein. Ongoing studies in this area may help determine calreticulin's function.

In addition to its localization to the lytic granules of cytotoxic T cells several observations implicate calreticulin, or calreticulin "family-members", in other facets of the immune response: (i) a peptide corresponding to the calreticulin leader sequence has been identified in the antigen-binding groove of class I molecules expressed by mutant cell lines;[31] (ii) mice immunized with irradiated melanoma cells produce antibodies against B50, a protein with an N-terminal amino acid sequence that is highly homologous to calreticulin;[18] (iii) the C1qR, which is expressed on B cells, neutrophils and endothelial cells, appears to be highly homologous to calreticulin.[19] In addition to binding C1q, the C1qR binds conglutinin, lung surfactant protein A and mannan binding protein.[19] Various cellular responses mediated by the ClqR have been described, including enhancement of phagocytosis, stimulation of oxygen radical generation and immunoglobulin secretion, and clearance of immune complexes from the circulation. Future definitive evidence that calreticulin and the C1qR are the same protein would contribute much to elucidation of the biological role of calreticulin.

Recent studies have also implicated calreticulin as an antigen in some pathological autoimmune responses, for example halothane hepatitis. Halothane hepatitis is a rare, often fatal, idiosyncratic reaction to the anesthetic halothane, which may have an immunological basis.[32,33] It appears that serum antibodies are directed against a number of liver microsomal proteins modified by the trifluoroacetyl halide metabolite of halothane,[34] and that calreticulin is one of these.[35] Serum antibodies from patients with halothane hepatitis reacted with both modified and native calreticulin to a greater extent than did serum antibodies from control patients.[35] Calreticulin is also a component of the human Ro/SS-A auto-antigen (Chapter 8).[14] This auto-antigen consists of at least four polypeptides which, as a complex, bind hYRNA molecules. It is thought that auto-antibodies produced against these proteins contribute to the tissue damage seen in patients with Sjörgren's syndrome and some forms of lupus erythematosus. Most interestingly, these auto-immune diseases often occur after cytomegalovirus infection, an infection which induces the expression of calreticulin.[36] Currently the significance of these observations is unknown. It is clear, however, that future work in these areas will prove invaluable in our efforts to determine the function(s) of calreticulin.

Perhaps the most surprising of recent findings is that calreticulin can inhibit steroid-sensitive gene expression (Chapter 6). In vitro, calreticulin inhibits steroid receptors from binding to their target DNA and, in vivo, it reduces their ability to enhance transcriptional activity (Chapter 6).[37,38] The most obvious question arising from these studies is how a protein resident in the endoplasmic reticulum can affect a steroid receptor found in either the cytosol or the nucleus. Are there cytosolic and/or nuclear forms of calreticulin? Trafficking studies in eukaryotic cells are required to determine whether or not calreticulin is targeted to the nucleus or found within the cytoplasm.

Recently Camacho and Lechleiter[39] made an exciting discovery while testing the role of calreticulin in $InsP_3$ mediated Ca^{2+} wave activity in *Xenopus* oocytes. Overexpression of the protein inhibited $InsP_3$ mediated repetitive Ca^{2+} waves.[39] Surprisingly, Ca^{2+} wave activity was also inhibited by overexpression of mutant which had a deletion high capacity Ca^{2+} binding (Ca^{2+} storage?) domain of calreticulin (C-domain)[39] (Chapter 2). These results demonstrated that calreticulin regulates intracellular Ca^{2+} signaling by a mechanism(s) that does not involve luminal Ca^{2+} storage. Camacho and Lechleiters[39] proposed that one of the physiological functions of calreticulin might be to prolong an $InsP_3$-induced rise in cytosolic Ca^{2+}. Furthermore, calreticulin may play an important function as a regulator of $InsP_3$ mediated intracellular Ca^{2+} signaling via a mechanism(s) that does not involve its high capacity Ca^{2+} binding/storage site.

The individual chapters of this book review some of the areas of study summarized above. As you read the book you will find many questions posed, along with current evidence and arguments. Is calreticulin a Ca^{2+} binding protein in vivo? What is the role of calreticulin in Ca^{2+} homeostasis? Does ion binding to calreticulin play some regulatory or signaling role, or is it required for protein stability? How does calreticulin affect steroid-sensitive gene expression and cell adhesion? Is calreticulin one of a new family of endoplasmic reticulum chaperones? Why is calreticulin so highly conserved throughout the animal kingdom?

From the cloning and localization of calreticulin to its ubiquitous distribution, this book explores the wide range of experimental observations that concern calreticulin. Certainly, this protein has sparked the interest of many investigators in many very diverse areas of research. Its high degree of conservation (Appendix A) throughout evolution is suggestive that it has an important cellular function. We hope that continued study of calreticulin will soon solve some of the intrigue, and clarify its role in the cell.

ACKNOWLEDGMENTS

Research in the authors laboratory is supported by the Medical Research Council of Canada, the Heart and Stroke Foundation of Alberta and the Muscular Dystrophy Association of Canada. M.M. is a Senior Scholar of the Alberta Heritage Foundation for Medical Research and MRC Scientist. We are grateful to R.E. Milner for critical reading of the manuscript.

REFERENCES

1. MacLennan DH, Campbell KP, Reithmeier RAF. Calsequestrin. In: Cheng WY, ed. Academic Press: Orlando, FL, 1983; 151-173.
2. Ostwald TJ, MacLennan DH. Isolation of a high affinity calcium binding protein from sarcoplasmic reticulum. J Biol Chem 1974; 249:974-979.
3. Michalak M, Campbell KP, MacLennan DH. Localization of the high affinity calcium binding protein and intrinsic glycoprotein in the sarcoplasmic reticulum membrane. J Biol Chem 1980; 255:1327-1334.
4. Waisman DM, Salimath BP, Anderson MJ. Isolation and characterization of CAB-63, a novel calcium-binding protein. J Biol Chem 1985; 260:1652-1660.
5. Khanna NC, Takuda M, Waisman DM. Conformational changes induced by binding of divalent cations to calregulin. J Biol Chem 1986; 261:8883-8887.

6. Khanna NC, Waisman DM. Development of a radioimmunoassay for quantitation of calregulin in bovine tissues. Biochemistry 1986; 25:1078-1082.

7. Khanna NC, Tokuda M, Waisman, DM. Comparison of calregulins from vertebrate livers. Biochem J 1987; 242:245-251.

8. Koch GLE. Reticuloplasmins: a novel group of proteins in the endoplasmic reticulum. J Cell Sci 1987; 87:491-492.

9. Smith MJ, Koch GLE. Multiple zones in the sequence of calreticulin (CRP55, calregulin, HACBP) a major calcium binding ER/SR proteins. EMBO J 1989; 8:3581-3586.

10. Fliegel L, Burns K, MacLennan DH et al. Molecular cloning of the high affinity calcium-binding protein (calreticulin) of skeletal muscle sarcoplasmic reticulum. J Biol Chem 1989; 264:21522-21528.

11. Fliegel L, Opas M, Michalak M. Identification of the high affinity calcium binding protein in muscle and non-muscle tissues. Biophys J 1988; Abstr. #338a.

12. Pelham HRB. Control of protein exit from the endoplasmic reticulumo Annu Rev Cell Biol 1989; 5:1-23.

13. Opas M, Fliegel L, Michalak M. Reticulin, a 55-kDa Ca-binding protein present in endoplasmic reticulum of many cell types. Fourth International Congress of Cell Biology, Montreal, Quebec, Canada, 1988; 353.

14. McCauliffe DP, Lux FA, Lieu TS et al. Molecular cloning, expression and chromosome 19 localization of human Ro autoantigen. J Clin Invest 1990; 85:1379-1391.

15. Murthy KK, Banville D, Srikant CB et al. Structural homology between the rat calreticulin gene product and the *Onchocerca volvulus* antigen Ral-1. Nucl Ac Res 1990; 18:4933.

16. Opas M, Dziak E, Fliegel L et al. Regulation of expression and intracellular distribution of calreticulin, a major calcium binding protein of nonmuscle cells. J Cell Physiol 1991; 149:160-171.

17. Dupuis M, Schaerer E, Krause KH et al. The calcium binding protein calreticulin is a major constituent of lytic granules in cytolytic T lymphocytes. J Exp Med 1993; 177:1-7.

18. Gersten DM, Bijwaard KE, Law LW et al. Homology of the B50 murine melanoma antigen to the Ro/SS-A antigen of human systemic lupus erythematosus and to calcium-binding proteins. Biochim Biophys Acta 1991; 1096:20-25.

19. Malhotra R, Willis AD, Jensenius JC et al. Structure and homology of human C1q receptor (collectin receptor). Immunol 1993; 78:341-348.

20. Sueyoshi T, McMullen BA, Marnell LL et al. A new procedure for separation of protein Z, prothrombin fragment 1.2 and calreticulin from human plasma. Throm Res 1991; 63:569-575.

21. Jaworski DC, Simmen FA, Lamoreaux W et al. A secreted calreticulin in ixodid tick saliva. J Insect Physiol 1995; 41:369-375.

22. Nakamura M, Moriya M, Baba T et al. An endoplasmic reticulum protein, calreticulin, is transported into the acrosome of rat sperm. Exp Cell Res 1993; 205:101-110.
23. Chen F, Hayes PM, Mulrooney DM et al. Identification and characterization of cDNA clones encoding plant calreticulin in barley. Plant Cell 1994; 6:835-843.
24. Denecke J, Carlsson LE, Vidal S et al. The tobacco homolog of mammalian calreticulin is present in protein complexes in vivo. Plant Cell 1995; 7:391-406.
25. Hossain A, Tagashira M, Hagiwara K et al. Is specific binding protein to Jaro spider toxin, a postsynaptic glutamate blocker, a family of calreticulin? Proc Jap Acad 1991; 67:203-208.
26. Conrad ME, Umbreit JN, Moore EG. Rat duodenal iron-binding protein mobilferrin is a homologue of calreticulin. Gastroenterology 1993; 104:1700-1704.
27. Neusfee WM, McCormick SJ, Clark RA. Calreticulin functions as a molecular chaperone in the biosynthesis of myeloperoxidase. J Biol Chem 1995; 270:4741-4747.
28. Nigam SK, Goldberg AL, Ho S et al. A set of endoplasmic reticulum proteins possessing properties of molecular chaperones includes Ca^{2+}-binding proteins and numbers of the thioredeoxin superfamily. J Biol Chem 1994; 269:1744-1749.
29. Kubawara K, Pinsky DJ, Schmidt AM et al. Calreticulin, an antithrombotic agent which binds to vitamin K-dependent coagulation factors, stimulates endothelial nitric oxide production, and limits thrombosis in canine coronary arteries. J Biol Chem 1995; 270:8179-8187.
30. Kennedy TE, Kuhl D, Barzilai A et al. Long-term sensitization training in *Aplysia* leads to an increase in calreticulin, a major presynaptic calcium-binding protein. Neuron 1992; 9:1013-1024.
31. Henderson RA, Michel H, Sakaguchi K et al. HLA-A2.1-associated peptides from mutant cell line: a second pathway of antigen presentation. Science 1992; 255:1264-1266
32. Neuberger J. Halothane and the liver-the present situation. J Clin Pharm Therap 1987; 12:269-271.
33. Pumford NR, Martin BM, Thomassen D et al. Serum antibodies from halothane hepatitis patients react with rat endoplasmic reticulum protein ERp72. Chem Res Toxicol 1993; 6:609-615.
34. Kenna JG, Neuberger J, Williams R. Identification by immunoblotting of three halothane-induced liver microsomal polypeptide antigens recognized by antibodies in sera from patients with halothane-associated hepatitis. J Pharmacol Exp Therap 1987; 242:733-740.
35. Butler LE, Thomassen D, Martin JL et al. The calcium binding protein calreticulin is covalently modified in rat liver by a reactive metabolite of the inhalation anesthetic halothane. Chem Res Toxicol 1992; 5:406-410.

36. Zhu JH, Newkirk MM. Viral induction of the human autoantigen calreticulin. Clin Invest Med 1994; 17:196-205.

37. Burns K, Duggan B, Atkinson EA et al. Modulation of gene expression by calreticulin binding to the glucocorticoid receptor. Nature 1994; 367:476-480.

38. Dedhar S, Rennie PS, Shago M et al. Inhibition of nuclear hormone receptor activity by calreticulin. Nature 1994; 367:480-483.

39. Camcho P, Lechleiter JD. Calreticulin inhibits repetitive intracellular Ca^{2+} waves. Cell 1995; 82:765-771.

BASIC CHARACTERISTICS AND ION BINDING TO CALRETICULIN

Shairaz Baksh and Marek Michalak

INTRODUCTION

Calreticulin is a protein that binds several different cations. In particular, this protein has been shown to have two distinct Ca^{2+} binding sites: a high capacity, low affinity site and a high affinity, low capacity site.[1,2] Because of its high capacity for Ca^{2+} binding (>20 moles of Ca^{2+}/mole of protein), it has been proposed that calreticulin may be a Ca^{2+} storage protein.[3] This possibility is reviewed, in detail, in Chapter 5. However, in addition to this potential role in Ca^{2+} storage, several other diverse functions have been proposed for calreticulin (see other chapters in this book).[4]

In this chapter we will review current knowledge on the structure of calreticulin. We will then discuss cation binding to calreticulin, including a review of i) how Ca^{2+} might be bound, ii) whether or not there are other cation binding site(s) on the protein, and iii) whether cation binding affects the "functional" properties of calreticulin. For amino acid sequence of calreticulin, the reader is referred to the Appendix at the end of this book.

THE STRUCTURE OF CALRETICULIN

AMINO ACID SEQUENCE

The amino acid sequence of rabbit skeletal muscle calreticulin is shown in Figure 2.1. A comparison of the amino acid sequences of different calreticulins is presented in the Appendix, which clearly

Calreticulin, edited by Marek Michalak. © 1996 R.G. Landes Company.

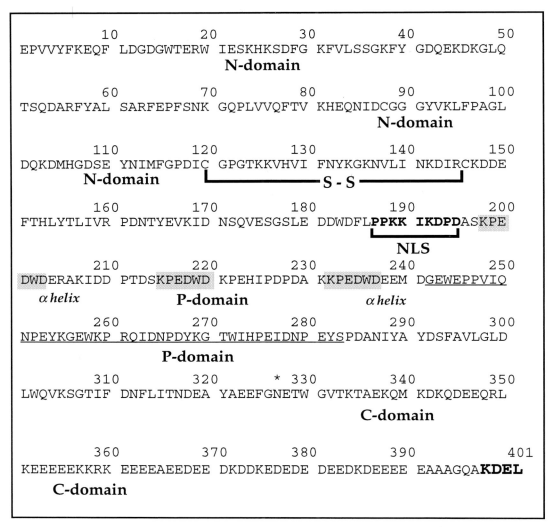

```
            10          20          30          40          50
EPVVYFKEQF  LDGDGWTERW  IESKHKSDFG  KFVLSSGKFY  GDQEKDKGLQ
                          N-domain

            60          70          80          90         100
TSQDARFYAL  SARFEPFSNK  GQPLVVQFTV  KHEQNIDCGG  GYVKLFPAGL
                                                  N-domain

           110         120         130         140         150
DQKDMHGDSE  YNIMFGPDIC  GPGTKKVHVI  FNYKGKNVLI  NKDIRCKDDE
        N-domain       └──────────── S - S ───────────┘

           160         170         180         190         200
FTHLYTLIVR  PDNTYEVKID  NSQVESGSLE  DDWDFLPPKK  IKDPDASKPE
                                         └─────────┘
                                              NLS

           210         220         230         240         250
DWDERAKIDD  PTDSKPEDWD  KPEHIPDPDA  KKPEDWDEEM  DGEWEPPVIQ
  α helix                P-domain                  α helix

           260         270         280         290         300
NPEYKGEWKP  RQIDNPDYKG  TWIHPEIDNP  EYSPDANIYA  YDSFAVLGLD
                        P-domain

           310         320       *  330         340         350
LWQVKSGTIF  DNFLITNDEA  YAEEFGNETW  GVTKTAEKQM  KDKQDEEQRL
                                                  C-domain

           360         370         380         390         401
KEEEEEKKRK  EEEEAEEDEE  DKDDKEDEDE  DEEDKDEEEE  EAAAGQAKDEL
     C-domain
```

Fig. 2.1. The amino acid sequence of rabbit skeletal muscle calreticulin. The amino acid sequence of rabbit skeletal muscle calreticulin was deduced from a nucleotide sequence.[6] The N-domain (residues 1 - 170), the P-domain (residues 187 - 285) and the C-domain (residues 286 - 401) are depicted. The location of the disulfide bond is indicated. The K-P-E-D-W-D repeat sequences (Fig. 2.2, Repeats A) are boxed. The region containing Repeats B (Fig. 2.2) is underlined. The putative nuclear localization signal (NLS) is shown. The asterisk at position 326 indicates a possible glycosylation site. The endoplasmic reticulum retention signal (KDEL) is shown in bold. The positions of predicted α-helical regions of the P-domain are indicated.

illustrates the marked degree of amino acid identity among the calreticulin sequences currently available. For example, there is over 90% amino acid identity among human, mouse, rat, rabbit and *Aplysia* calreticulins. Furthermore, the sequence of plant calreticulin exhibits over 50% amino acid identity when compared with the animal protein (Appendix). For mammalian calreticulins, this high degree of sequence identity is also observed in the nucleotide sequence of the cDNAs that encode the protein. In addition to being highly conserved, calreticulin also appears to be a ubiquitous protein which may play an essential role in cell biology.[3]

The calculated molecular weight of rabbit calreticulin is 46,567 daltons. However, when analyzed by SDS-PAGE (pH 8.0 Laemmli system), calreticulin migrates with an apparent molecular weight of 60,000-63,000 daltons.[5] This discrepancy is probably related to the high number of negatively charged amino acids found at the carboxyl-terminal (C-terminal) of the protein. Hydropathy plots of calreticulin reveal a hydrophobic N-terminal signal sequence (confirmed by in vitro translation of mRNA encoding rabbit, and human γ, calreticulin)[6,7] but no potential transmembrane segments.[3] Mature calreticulin contains 109 acidic and 52 basic amino acids and has a pI value of 4.46 (Fig. 2.1). Structural predictions for calreticulin suggest that it has at least three domains (see below).[6,8] The first half of the molecule forms a globular domain; this is followed by a proline-rich sequence containing specific amino acid repeats (Repeat A and Repeat B, Fig. 2.2), and then by the carboxyl-terminus, which contains thirty-seven acidic residues. Interestingly, the highest degree of amino acid identity between different calreticulins is in the amino-terminal (N-terminal) half of the molecule.

Different functional motifs or consensus sequences within the amino acid sequence of calreticulin have been noted. For example, calreticulin has two lysosome targeting signals (residues 42-48 and 347-353). Note, however, that the protein has not been localized to this intracellular compartment. Calreticulin also contains PEST regions (rich in proline, glutamic acid, serine and/or threonine) which are thought to make a protein susceptible to rapid intracellular degradation. Again, it is not clear whether these are functional. The protein also contains a nuclear localization signal (residues 187-195: Fig. 2.1), and myristylation, amidation and heparin binding sites, none of which has been proven to have functional

Repeat A

Consensus: P-x-x-I-P-D-P-x-A-x-K-P-E-D-W-D-E

CRT
- A1: 188 P-K-K-I-K-D-P-D-A-S-K-P-E-D-W-D-E 204
- A2: 205 R-A-K-I-D-D-P-T-D-S-K-P-E-D-W-D-K 221
- A3: 222 P-E-H-I-P-D-P-D-A-K-K-P-E-D-W-D-E 238

CNX
- A1: 275 S-R-E-I-E-D-P-E-D-R-K-P-E-D-W-D-E 290
- A2: 291 R-P-K-I-P-D-P-E-A-V-K-P-D-D-W-D-E 307
- A3: 310 P-A-K-I-P-D-E-E-A-T-K-P-E-G-W-L-D 326
- A4: 329 P-E-Y-V-P-D-P-A-E-K-P-E-D-W-D-E 345

CMG
- A1: 265 P-R-E-I-A-D-P-S-D-K-K-P-F-E-W-D-D 281
- A2: 281 R-A-K-I-P-D-P-T-A-V-K-P-E-D-W-D-E 297
- A3: 300 P-A-Q-I-E-D-S-S-A-V-K-P-D-G-W-L-D 316
- A4: 319 P-K-F-I-P-N-P-K-A-E-K-P-E-D-W-S-D 335

CNE-1
- A1: 228 P-L-M-I-P-D-V-S-V-A-K-P-H-D-W-D-D 244
- A2: 245 R-I-R-I-P-D-P-E-A-V-K-L-S-D-R-D-E 261
- A3: 264 P-L-M-I-P-H-P-D-G-T-E-P-P-E-W-N-S 280
- A4: 283 P-E-Y-I-L-D-P-N-A-Q-K-P-S-W-W-K-E 299

CNE-2
- A1: 239 P-V-E-I-Y-D-P-E-D-I-K-P-A-D-W-V-D 255
- A2: 256 E-P-E-I-P-D-P-N-A-V-K-P-D-D-W-D-E 272
- A3: 275 P-R-M-I-P-D-P-D-A-V-K-P-E-D-W-L-E 291
- A4: 294 P-L-Y-I-I-P-D-P-E-A-Q-K-P-E-D-W-D-D 310

Repeat B

Consensus: G-E-W-x-P-P-x-I-x-N-P-x-Y-x

CRT
- B1: 242 G-E-W-E-P-P-V-I-Q-N-P-E-Y-K 255
- B2: 256 G-E-W-K-P-R-Q-I-D-N-P-D-Y-K 269
- B3: 270 G-T-W-I-H-P-E-I-D-N-P-E-Y-S 283

CNX
- B1: 349 G-E-W-E-A-P-Q-I-A-N-P-K-C-E 362
- B2: 368 G-V-W-Q-R-P-M-I-D-N-P-N-Y-K 380
- B3: 382 G-K-W-K-P-M-I-D-N-P-N-Y-Q 395
- B4: 396 G-I-W-K-P-R-I-P-N-P-D-F-F 409

CMG
- B1: 339 G-E-W-A-E-P-H-I-P-N-P-D-C-Q 352
- B2: 356 G-E-W-K-P-M-I-D-N-P-K-Y-K 370
- B3: 371 G-I-W-R-P-M-I-N-N-P-N-Y-Q 384
- B4: 385 G-L-W-S-P-Q-K-I-P-N-P-D-Y-F 398

CNE-1
- B1: 303 G-E-W-I-P-M-I-K-N-P-L-C-T 316
- B2: 322 G-Q-Q-I-P-G-L-I-N-A-K-Y-K 335
- B3: 338 G-E-L-N-E-I-I-N-P-N-Y-M-G-E 351
- B4: 349 G-E-W-H-I-P-P-E-I-E-N-P-L-Y 362

CNE-2
- B1: 314 G-D-W-I-P-S-E-I-I-N-P-K-C-I 327
- B2: 333 G-E-W-K-P-M-I-R-N-P-N-Y-R 346
- B3: 347 G-P-W-S-P-M-I-P-N-P-E-F-I 360
- B4: 361 G-E-W-Y-P-R-K-I-P-N-P-D-Y-F 374

significance. Importantly calreticulin contains a C-terminal KDEL (or HDEL) amino acid sequence[9] which is responsible for its retention in the lumen of the endoplasmic reticulum.[10]

Finally, two distinct, short amino acid sequences within calreticulin are repeated, in triplicate, in the central, proline-rich region of the protein (Fig. 2.2). The functional significance of these sequence repeats is not proven; however, recent experiments indicate that the repeats of Type A may be involved in the high affinity binding of Ca^{2+} to calreticulin (see below). Repeats of Type A and B are also found in proteins similar to calreticulin, for example calnexin[5] and calmegin[11] (Fig. 2.2) and they might also play a role in Ca^{2+} binding to these proteins.

GLYCOSYLATION

Calreticulin contains a consensus site for N-linked glycosylation, at residue 326 (Fig. 2.1). This site is conserved in human, rabbit, mouse, rat, *Xenopus, Aplysia* and bovine calreticulin, but not in the *Drosophila*, tick, plant and nematode protein (Appendix). Bovine brain and *Schistosoma mansoni* calreticulins have an additional amino acid consensus sequence for glycosylation, at residue 162 (Appendix).[12] While no carbohydrate has been detected in calreticulin from human, mouse, rabbit, rat sperm, dog, or chicken liver (Appendix), calreticulin from bovine liver and brain, rat liver, and chinese hamster ovary (CHO) cells has been shown to be glycosylated.[3,12-14] The glycosylation pattern of *Schistosoma mansoni* calreticulin, which contains the two potential glycosylation sites, has not been investigated.

Bovine liver calreticulin binds to a Concanavalin A affinity column.[14] Using glycopeptidase F digestion and electrospray ionization mass spectroscopy, Matsuoka et al[12] identified a high mannose sugar structure (composition $(GlcNAc)_2Man_5$) in bovine brain calreticulin. This is a typical composition for glycoproteins of the endoplasmic reticulum. The carbohydrate was found at Asn162, the site unique, so far, to the bovine brain and *Schistosoma mansoni* proteins. In neither case was glycosylation of Asn326 observed.

Fig. 2.2. (left) *Conserved amino acid sequences repeat in calreticulin. The consensus sequences of amino acids in Repeats A and B of the P-domain of calreticulin are shown. Repeats A and B are also found in calnexin, calmegin and yeast calnexins. x, denotes any amino acid. CRT, rabbit skeletal muscle calreticulin;[6] CNX, canine calnexin;[28] CMG, calmegin;[11] CNE-1, S. cerevisiae calnexin;[44,45] CNE-2, S. pombe calnexin.[46]*

Rat liver calreticulin contains a complex hybrid type of oligosaccharide, with a terminal galactose residue.[13] This type of glycosylation is rather unusual for proteins resident in the endoplasmic reticulum, and, in fact, the terminal galactose indicates that the protein must pass through the trans-Golgi before being transported back to the endoplasmic reticulum. In keeping with this, Söling's group has shown that this terminal galactosylation is abolished when vesicular transport from the intermediate- to the trans-Golgi is blocked.[14]

To date, the evidence available indicates that glycosylation of calreticulin is species and/or tissue specific. Nevertheless, an exciting observation made recently, by Jethmalani et al,[15] suggests that calreticulin may undergo stress-induced glycosylation. These authors found that one of the proteins undergoing major glycosylation, as a result of heat-shock in CHO cells, was calreticulin (they originally identified the protein as P-GS67). The role for this glycosylation of calreticulin is not known.

DISULFIDE BRIDGE

Calreticulin has three highly conserved cysteine residues at positions 88, 120 and 146 (App. A). Bovine brain calreticulin has one intramolecular disulfide bridge, Cys120-Cys146 (Fig. 2.1).[12] A disulfide bridge has also been identified in calreticulins from human placenta[16] and rabbit (Baksh and Michalak, unpublished observation). It is likely that all calreticulins have this disulfide bridge, which may play a role in maintaining proper folding of the N-terminal region of the protein.

PHOSPHORYLATION

Calreticulin has multiple copies of the recognition sequences for several protein kinases, including protein kinase C (clustered at the N-terminal region of the protein: residues 17-19, 36-38, 61-63, 68-70, 79-81 and 124-126), casein kinase II (residues 51-54, 172-175, 178-181, 196-200, 204-208, 307-311, and 316-319) and tyrosine kinase (residues 261-268). Despite these consensus sequences we have found that neither canine pancreatic calreticulin, nor recombinant calreticulin, are phosphorylated, in vitro, by protein kinase C, cAMP-dependent protein kinase, casein kinase II or tyrosine kinase (Michalak et al, unpublished observations). Calreticulin also has an amino acid sequence with marked similarity to the active site of protein kinase C (215-224: K-P-E-D-W-D-K-P-E-H). However, the protein does not contain the consensus amino acid sequence GxGxxG found in the ATP binding motif of all protein kinases. Furthermore, using histone III as a substrate for protein kinase C phosphorylation, we were unable to detect any protein kinase activity in calreticulin. However, Singh et al[17] have found that calreticulin undergoes autophosphorylation, in Vero 76 cells, and that this phosphorylation is essential for an interaction between calreticulin and the 3' *cis*-acting element of rubella virus RNA (see Chapter 7). Serine and threonine residues within the N-terminal half of the protein were phosphorylated. In these studies the degree of phosphorylation of calreticulin increased as a result of the viral infection, without a concomitant change in protein levels.

NUCLEIC ACID BINDING SITES

Nakhasi's group[17] has identified calreticulin as a binding protein for rubella virus RNA. This property of calreticulin is described in detail in Chapter 7. Although calreticulin does not have the conventional ribonucleoprotein (RNP) binding motif found in many nuclear and cytoplasmic RNA binding proteins, residues 3-6 of calreticulin (A-V-Y-F) are present in the RNA recognition motif of human splicing factor ASF/SF2.[17] The autophosphorylation of calreticulin, discussed above, and the phosphorylation-dependent interaction of calreticulin with nucleic acids may be physiologically relevant. In particular, their possible significance in the pathology of autoimmune diseases is discussed in Chapter 8.

THE THREE DIMENSIONAL STRUCTURE OF CALRETICULIN

It has been proposed that calreticulin can be divided into three structurally distinct domains.[3,8] A hypothetical model of these three domains is shown in Figure 2.3.

N-domain

The first domain, which encompasses the N-terminal half of the molecule (residues 1-170), is predicted to be a highly folded, globular structure,[8] containing 8 anti-parallel β-strands connected by protein loops (N-domain) (Fig. 2.3). Two regions of short α-helices are predicted at residues 98-103 and 149-154. This domain has an approximately neutral net charge and is the region of

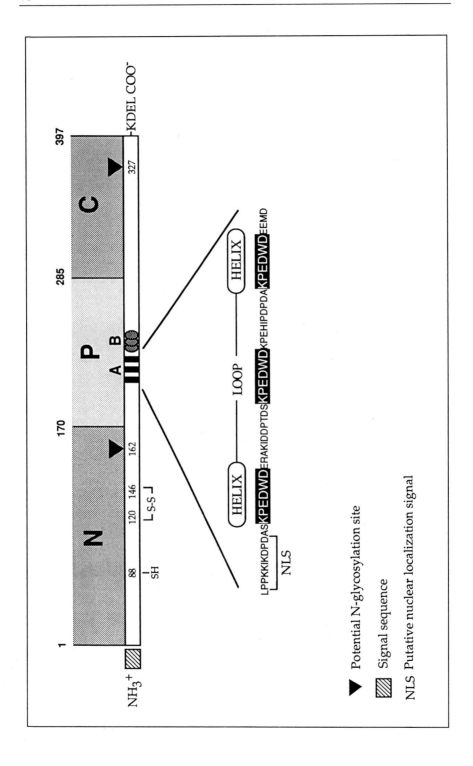

calreticulin responsible for the protein's interaction with the DNA binding domain of steroid receptors (Chapter 6), Zn^{2+} binding properties (unpublished observations), rubella virus RNA binding (Chapter 7), and interaction with the α-subunit of integrin.[18,19]

P-domain

The middle portion of calreticulin comprises a proline-rich sequence (P-domain) containing 16 mol% proline residues which are spaced every four or five amino acids (residues 187-285). This domain contains 18 of the 25 proline residues, and 6 of the 11 tryptophan residues, found within calreticulin. The first part of the P-domain is highly charged and contains two sets of repeat sequences (Fig. 2.3). There are three repeats of the amino acid sequence P-x-x-I-x-D-P-D-A-x-K-P-E-D-W-D-E (Repeat A, Fig. 2.2) followed by three repeats of the sequence G-x-W-x-P-P-x-I-x-N-P-x-Y-x (Repeat B, Fig. 2.2). The region of calreticulin containing the first set of repeats (Repeats A) may be responsible for high affinity Ca^{2+} binding to the protein (unpublished results).[20] The second portion of the P-domain comprises a proline-, serine-, and threonine-rich sequence (residues 246-316) which is predicted to contain a repeating, rigid turn structure separating the globular head of the protein from the acidic tail.

C-domain

The C-terminal quarter of the protein (the C-domain) is highly acidic and highly negatively charged. Of the last 57 residues within the C-domain, 37 are aspartic or glutamic acid. The acidic amino acid residues are organized in polyacidic stretches that are flanked by basic residues. Chemical modification of these basic residues reduces the capacity of this region to bind Ca^{2+}.[21] The C-domain of calreticulin, which has the most divergent amino acid sequence (appendix), terminates with the KDEL endoplasmic reticulum retention sequence (Fig. 2.3). This domain is responsible for the interaction of calreticulin with a set of endoplasmic/sarcoplasmic reticulum proteins[22] and with blood clotting factors (Chapter 10).

---

*Fig. 2.3. (left) The domain structure of calreticulin. A putative model of calreticulin domains is shown. The N-domain (**N**) and the C-domain (**C**) contain potential glycosylation sites. The N-domain contains three cysteine residues including one disulfide bridge. Location of Repeats A (**A**) and Repeats B (**B**) in the P-domain (**P**) is depicted. A section containing Repeats A and a putative "helix-loop-helix" Ca^{2+} binding region are magnified.*

PROTEINS SIMILAR TO CALRETICULIN

Calreticulin belongs to the family of KDEL proteins that are resident in the endoplasmic reticulum. It is not surprising, therefore, that the amino acid sequence of calreticulin has some similarity to the amino acid sequences of other lumenal endoplasmic reticulum proteins, including protein disulfide isomerase (PDI), immunoglobulin binding proteins (BiP, Grp78), ERp72, endoplasmin (Grp94), and ERp61.[23] These proteins all contain a relatively large proportion of acidic amino acid residues (generally clustered at the C-terminus) and have a hydrophobic, N-terminal, endoplasmic reticulum signal sequence. They all also contain either the C-terminal KDEL endoplasmic reticulum retention sequence, or the related sequences KEEL (ERp72) and QEDL (ERp61).[9,24,25]

Calsequestrin, a major Ca^{2+} binding protein of muscle sarcoplasmic reticulum membranes,[21] has similar physicochemical properties to calreticulin. Both proteins are highly acidic and have characteristically large Ca^{2+} binding capacities. They both also stain blue with the cationic carbocyanine dye Stains-All, and have an electrophoretic mobility on SDS-PAGE which is highly pH-sensitive.[26] Some antibodies raised against muscle calsequestrin also recognize calreticulin, leading to some earlier reports describing calreticulin as a calsequestrin-like protein.[3] However, although the overall amino acid composition of these proteins is similar,[26] the amino acid sequences of calsequestrin and calreticulin are very different; the two proteins share less than 10% amino acid identity.

In contrast, there are three proteins known to share significant amino acid similarities with calreticulin: RAL-1 (*Onchocerca* calreticulin), calnexin and calmegin. RAL-1 is an antigen found in patients with symptomatic features of onchocerciasis (river blindness). Cloning of this antigen revealed that the protein is similar to mammalian calreticulin (Appendix).[27] The first 300 amino acids display marked amino acid sequence identity, especially in the central, proline-rich region of calreticulin. The area of least homology is at the C-terminus. In contrast with calreticulin, the C-terminal region of RAL-1 is positively, rather than negatively, charged and does not terminate with the KDEL amino acid sequence.[27] These differences support the suggestion that, unlike calreticulin, RAL-1 would not bind Ca^{2+} with high capacity and would not be retained in the lumen of the endoplasmic reticulum. The precise functional significance, and role in the pathology of onchocerciasis, of this protein is not clear at present. It also remains to be determined whether or not *Onchocerca* expresses a conventional calreticulin.

Calnexin is an endoplasmic reticular chaperone. Recently, mammalian, plant, nematode and yeast cDNAs encoding calnexin have been isolated and the protein amino acid sequences deduced from the nucleotide sequences.[28] The sequences reveal that calnexin shares several regions of similarity with calreticulin, ranging from 42% to 78% identity.[28] Interestingly, several of the distinctive sequences that are highly conserved among different calreticulins are present in calnexin. The most striking of these are the Repeats A (Fig. 2.2) and B (Fig. 2.2) found in the P-domain of calreticulin, both of which are present in calnexin.[28] This region of both proteins may be involved in Ca^{2+} binding.[29] Although the C-terminal regions of both proteins are highly acidic, this region of calnexin is predicted to be extracytoplasmic.[28] The sequence similarity between calnexin and calreticulin suggests that these proteins may have some functional properties in common (Chapter 4). Calnexin, which associates with several different multimeric protein complexes, including MHC 1 heavy chain, the T-cell receptor and membrane immunoglobulin, has been shown to have chaperone activity.[30] Interestingly, a chaperone function for calreticulin has recently been documented (Chapter 4).[31,32]

Calmegin is a novel Ca^{2+}-binding protein that is expressed specifically during meiotic germ cell development, and not in other, somatic tissues.[11] The amino acid sequence of calmegin exhibits >58% similarity to calnexin and a partial similarity to calreticulin. Again, the highest degree of similarity between calmegin and calreticulin is in the central region of calreticulin (P-domain, see below). Particularly, four copies of the characteristic amino acid repeats A and B are also present in calmegin[11] (Fig. 2.2). Calmegin is synthesized with a hydrophobic signal sequence and is associated with the endoplasmic reticulum, but it does not terminate with a KDEL retention signal.[11] The function of calmegin has not been determined, but it may play a role in the control of Ca^{2+} homeostasis during meiotic germ cell development.

Some proteins appear to have blocks of sequence identical to calreticulin followed by blocks of completely unrelated sequence.[30] For example, in C1qR, nine of twelve peptides were found to have identical amino acid sequences to portions of calreticulin.[30] Two remaining peptides were found to be similar to calreticulin, and a final peptide was not present in calreticulin.[30] Not surprisingly, the amino acid composition of the C1qR is very similar to that of calreticulin, but slight differences have also been identified. Specifically, the cysteine content was found to be slightly higher in the C1qR than in calreticulin (3% compared with 1%). Another protein which appears to be related to calreticulin/C1qR has been isolated from human spleen.[30] This protein migrates in SDS-PAGE at the same mobility as C1qR, has an identical N-terminal amino acid sequence and is recognized by anti C1qR and anti Ro/SS-A antibodies, but, intriguingly, has a different overall charge than C1qR–Ro/SS-A.[30]

Another protein exhibiting this unusual sequence homology with calreticulin was recently isolated from bovine brain.[33] The pI, amino acid composition and immunological characteristics of this protein are very similar to those of calreticulin, but the N-terminal amino acid sequence differs.[33] Recently a cDNA clone has been obtained which may encode this protein.[33] The protein encoded is of 387 amino acids, with a possible signal sequence of 34 amino acids and a C-terminal KDEL tetrapeptide.[33] The deduced sequence for the C-terminal 318 amino acids is highly similar to mouse calreticulin, but a block of 69 amino acids at the N-terminus is completely divergent. In Northern blots, a 3.75 kilobase mRNA species was detected by a cDNA probe encoding this divergent region.[33] Interestingly, a similarly sized transcript that hybridized with calreticulin cDNA has been detected in previous studies by Northern blot analysis of mRNA from fast- and slow-twitch muscles.[6] In both cases, a cDNA corresponding to the 3.75 kilobase mRNA has not yet been isolated. However, the available evidence supports the suggestion that the 3.75 kilobase mRNA might be a transcript for an isoform of calreticulin.

THE CATION BINDING PROPERTIES OF CALRETICULIN

CALCIUM BINDING

Calreticulin has two Ca^{2+} binding sites: a high affinity, low capacity site ($K_d = 1$ μM; $B_{max} = 1$ mole Ca^{2+}/mole protein) and a low affinity high capacity sites ($K_d = 2$ mM; $B_{max} = 20$ moles Ca^{2+}/mole protein).[1,2] The location of these two sites within the protein has been mapped by expressing various domains of calreticulin in *E. coli*.[2] The functional significance of Ca^{2+} binding to calreticulin is not yet clear. Indeed, in vitro studies have yielded conflicting results. For example, interaction between calreticulin and the DNA binding domain of the glucocorticoid receptor is Ca^{2+} independent. Yet, binding of the protein to the K-G-L-F-F-K-R peptide, found in the α subunit of integrin, is Ca^{2+} dependent. Calreticulin binds to a set of low molecular weight proteins of endoplasmic and sarcoplasmic reticulum, and these interactions are not Ca^{2+} dependent. However, interactions between calreticulin and denatured polypeptides might be Ca^{2+}-dependent.[31]

THE HIGH CAPACITY CA^{2+} BINDING SITE

The low affinity, high capacity Ca^{2+} binding is localized to the carboxyl-terminal region (C-domain) of calreticulin (Fig. 2.4). This domain consists of clusters of aspartic and glutamic acid residues which are likely involved in the Ca^{2+} binding (Fig. 2.1). This is in keeping with observations that several other Ca^{2+} binding proteins have clusters of acidic amino acid residues which are implicated in their Ca^{2+} binding behavior, for example, chromogranin A and

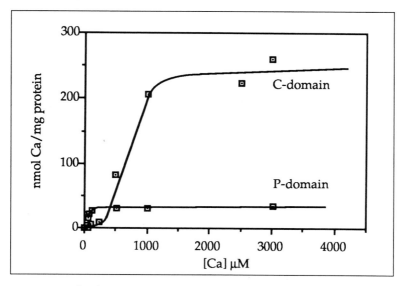

Fig. 2.4. Ca^{2+} binding to the P- and C-domains of calreticulin.[43] Ca^{2+} binding to GST-fusion proteins was carried out by equilibrium dialysis.[2] Reproduced with permission from Baksh S, Michalak M. J Biol Chem 1991; 266:21458-21465.

skeletal and cardiac muscle calsequestrin.[34] The C-domain of calreticulin also binds Mg^{2+}, but the physiological significance of this observation has yet to be determined. The possibility that high capacity Ca^{2+} binding to calreticulin may play a role in Ca^{2+} storage in the lumen of the endoplasmic/sarcoplasmic reticulum is discussed in detail in Chapter 5. In addition, other functions for the high capacity Ca^{2+} binding have been suggested, including the possibility that calreticulin may be a "carrier" of Ca^{2+} for specific cellular processes regulated by Ca^{2+}. For example, the protein has been localized to the neurons of the marine mollusk, *Aplysia californica*, where it appears to be associated with long term memory.[35] Calreticulin is also found in the acrosomal body of spermatozoa and spermatids where it might be involved in delivering a Ca^{2+} signal during the fertilization process.[36] The protein also appears to play some role in: i) the penetration of the skin by cercariae of *Schistosoma mansoni;*[37-39] ii) the blood coagulation cascade (Chapter 10); and iii) the killing activity of perforin molecules in cytotoxic T cells (Chapter 9).

The High Affinity Ca^{2+} Binding Site

This Ca^{2+} binding site is located within the P-domain of calreticulin (Fig. 2.4), and binds approximately 1 mole of Ca^{2+}/mole of protein with a dissociation constant of 1-6 μM. The functional significance of this high affinity Ca^{2+} binding site remains to be elucidated. For it to be physiologically relevant, the free concentration of Ca^{2+} in the lumen of the endoplasmic reticulum would have to be approximately 1 μM (Chapter 5). The site could play a regulatory role, allowing calreticulin to modulate, in a Ca^{2+}-dependent manner, the activity of other endoplasmic reticulum proteins.

Functionally, the most clearly understood high affinity Ca^{2+} binding proteins are members of the EF-hand family, in which Ca^{2+} binding frequently plays a regulatory role.[40] However, the amino acid sequence of calreticulin does not contain an EF-hand consensus sequence (Fig. 2.1). Nevertheless, secondary structure analysis has revealed that the P-domain may contain a helix-turn-helix motif reminiscent of the secondary structure of the EF-hand.[40] This implies that calreticulin may contain a novel motif for high affinity Ca^{2+} binding.

Recent studies in our laboratory have revealed that high affinity Ca^{2+} binding to calreticulin is localized to the Repeat A region of the P-domain (Fig. 2.2 and 2.3). These results are in keeping with the results of an earlier analysis of Ca^{2+} binding to calnexin.[29] Calnexin contains four of the Repeats A and B, three of which are identical to those found in calreticulin (Fig. 2.2). Tjoelker et al[29] showed that a recombinant peptide, encompassing amino acids 254 -334 of calnexin (P-domain) and containing only Repeat A, was sufficient to bind Ca^{2+}. In further studies, using fusion proteins, we have also found that there is a strict requirement for both the first and third Repeat A (Fig. 2.1) in order to form the high affinity Ca^{2+} binding site (Baksh and Michalak, unpublished data). Together these results suggest that the Repeat B is not directly involved in Ca^{2+} binding; however, it may be required to stabilize the conformation of the Ca^{2+} binding site.

ZINC BINDING

Waisman's group has determined that calreticulin also binds 14 moles of Zn^{2+}/mole of protein, with relatively low affinity (~300 μM).[41] The binding of Zn^{2+} to calreticulin induces dramatic conformational changes in the protein which can be measured by changes in its intrinsic fluorescence, its circular dichroism spectrum, and its interaction with phenyl-Sepharose beads.[41,42] Since calreticulin does not contain a consensus sequence for a "Zn^{2+}-finger", the location of the Zn^{2+} binding was difficult to predict. In recent studies we have found that calreticulin may have two distinct Zn^{2+} binding sites; a high affinity site ($K_d = 0.8$ μM; $B_{max} = 26$ moles Zn^{2+}/mole protein) localized within the globular N-domain of the protein, and a lower affinity site ($K_d = 47.6$ μM; $B_{max} = 83$ moles Zn^{2+}/mole protein) (unpublished observations). Physiological concentrations of Ca^{2+} and Mg^{2+} compete with Zn^{2+} binding to this second site, suggesting that it may not be physiologically relevant. In contrast, the high affinity Zn^{2+} binding site is localized to the N-domain of calreticulin, a region of the protein that binds neither Ca^{2+} nor Mg^{2+}. Since this region of calreticulin interacts with the DNA binding domain of steroid receptors (Chapter 6), the rubella virus RNA (Chapter 7) and the α-subunit of integrin, the Zn^{2+} binding could play a role in modulation of these interactions. Alternatively, calreticulin could play a role in the regulation of intracellular levels of Zn^{2+}.

IRON BINDING

Mobilferrin, located in the rat duodenum, is an iron binding protein (K_d = 90 μM; B_{max} = 1 mole Fe^{3+}/mole protein). In addition to iron, this protein binds other metals (zinc>cobalt>copper>lead). It has been proposed that mobilferrin may be responsible for the movement of iron into non-intestinal cells, which do not contain the transferrin receptors that normally function in the uptake of iron. Conrad et al[22] have shown recently that mobilferrin has an N-terminal amino acid sequence identical to calreticulin. Furthermore, anti-mobilferrin antibodies cross-react with calreticulin. These two observations suggest that mobilferrin and calreticulin may be the same protein. Interestingly, mobilferrin was also found to be associated with integrins.[22] This is consistent with the observation that calreticulin binds to the α-subunit of integrin and modulates adhesion-dependent signaling (to be physiologically relevant, this function would require that calreticulin also be localized to the cytoplasm).[18,19] Molecular cloning of mobilferrin will clarify whether these two proteins are indeed identical.

ARE THERE ANY FUNCTIONAL CONSEQUENCES OF CA²⁺ BINDING TO CALRETICULIN?

What is the role of Ca^{2+} binding to calreticulin? The most logical function of Ca^{2+} binding to calreticulin is to store Ca^{2+}. This function of calreticulin would provide cells with "reservoir" of intracellular Ca^{2+} to carry out a variety of Ca^{2+}-dependent processes without having to relay on the availability of the extracellular Ca^{2+}. Indeed, the protein was proposed to play a Ca^{2+} storage role in the endoplasmic reticulum and perhaps in other intracellular organelles (granules, nuclear envelope) but this function has not yet been documented in vivo (Chapter 5). Is Ca^{2+} binding to calreticulin critical for the many other functions proposed for the protein? At present, it is rather difficult to answer this important question. Interaction between calreticulin and the DNA binding domain of the glucocorticoid receptor is Ca^{2+} independent. Yet, binding of the protein to the K-G-L-F-F-K-R peptide, found in the α subunit of integrin, is Ca^{2+} dependent. Calreticulin binds to a set of low molecular weight proteins of endoplasmic and sarcoplasmic reticulum. These interactions are not Ca^{2+} dependent. However, interactions between calreticulin and denatured polypeptides might be Ca^{2+}-dependent.[31] Hopefully, in the near future, we will have a better understanding of the functional consequences of Ca^{2+} binding (and/or other cation) to calreticulin. It would be fascinating to understand a role for the unique high affinity Ca^{2+} binding site in the protein.

ACKNOWLEDGMENT

We are grateful to Thidi (Dr. M. Waser) for designing the figures. We thank Dr. R.E. Milner for critical reading of the manuscript. Research in the authors' laboratory is supported by the Medical Research Council of Canada, the Heart and Stroke Foundation of Alberta and the Muscular Dystrophy Association of Canada. M.M. is a Senior Scholar of the Alberta Heritage Foundation for Medical Research and MRC Scientist. S.B. was a recipient of a studentship from the Heart and Stroke Foundation of Canada.

REFERENCES

1. Ostwald TJ, MacLennan DH. Isolation of a high affinity calcium binding protein from sarcoplasmic reticulum. J Biol Chem 1974; 249:974-979.
2. Baksh S, Michalak M. Expression of calreticulin in *Escherichia coli* and identification of its Ca^{2+} binding domains. J Biol Chem 1991; 266:21458-21465.
3. Michalak M, Milner RE, Burns K, Opas M. Calreticulin. Biochem J 1992; 285:681-692.
4. Nash PD, Opas M, Michalak M. Calreticulin: not just another calcium binding protein. Mol Cell Biochem 1994; 135:71-78.
5. Milner RE, Baksh S, Shemanko C et al. Calreticulin, and not calsequestrin, is the major calcium binding protein of smooth muscle sarcoplasmic reticulum and liver endoplasmic reticulum. J Biol Chem 1991; 266:7155-7165.
6. Fliegel L, Burns K, MacLennan DH et al. Molecular cloning of the high affinity calcium-binding protein (calreticulin) of skeletal muscle sarcoplasmic reticulum. J Biol Chem 1989; 264:21522-21528.
7. Rokeach LA, Haselby JA, Meilof JF et al. Characterization of the autoantigen calreticulin. J Immunol 1991; 147:3031-3039.
8. Smith MJ, Koch GLE. Multiple zones in the sequence of calreticulin (CRP55, calregulin, HACBP) a major calcium binding ER/SR protein. EMBO J 1989; 8:3581-3586.
9. Pelham HRB. Control of protein exit from the endoplasmic reticulum. Annu Rev Cell Biol 1989; 5:1-23.

10. Sönnichsen B, Füllekrug J, Van PN et al. Retention and retrieval: both mechanisms cooperate to maintain calreticulin in the endoplasmic reticulum. J Cell Sci 1994; 107:2705-2717.

11. Watanabe D, Yamada K, Nishina Y et al. Molecular cloning of a novel Ca^{2+}-binding protein (calmegin) specifically expressed during male meiotic germ cell development. J Biol Chem 1994; 269:7744-7749.

12. Matsuoka K, Seta K, Yamakawa Y et al. Covalent structure of bovine brain calreticulin. Biochem J 1994; 298:435-442.

13. Waisman DM, Salimath BP, Anderson MJ. Isolation and characterization of CAB-63, a novel calcium-binding protein. J Biol Chem 1985; 260:1652-1660.

14. Van PN, Peter F, Söling H-D. Four intracisternal calcium-binding glycoproteins from rat liver microsomes with high affinity for calcium. J Biol Chem 1989; 264:17494-17501.

15. Jethmalani SM, Henle KJ, Kaushal GP. Heat shock-induced prompt glycosylation. Identification of P-SG67 as calreticulin. J Biol Chem 1994; 269:23603-23609.

16. Houen G, Koch C. Human placenta calreticulin: purification, characterization and association with other proteins. Acta Chem Scand 1994; 48:905-911.

17. Singh NK, Rouault TA, Liu TY et al. Calreticulin is an RNA binding phosphoprotein which interacts with the 3'*cis*-acting element of rubella virus RNA. Proc Natl Acad Sci USA 1994; 91:12770-12774

18. Rojiani MV, Finlay BB, Gray V et al. In vitro interaction of a polypeptide homologous to human Ro/SS-A antigen (calreticulin) with a highly conserved amino acid sequence in the cytoplasmic domain of integrin α subunits. Biochemistry 1991; 30:9859-9865.

19. Leung-Hagesteijn CY, Milankov K, Michalak M et al. Integrin-mediated cell attachment to extracellular matrix substrates is inhibited upon downregulation of expression of calreticulin, an intracellular integrin α-subunit binding protein. J Cell Sci 1994; 107:589-600.

20. Peter FP, Van NP, Söling H-D. Different sorting of Lys-Asp-Glu-Leu proteins in rat liver. J Biol Chem 1992; 267:10631-10637.

21. MacLennan DH, Campbell KP, Reithmeier RAF. Calsequestrin. In: Cheng WY, ed. Academic Press: Orlando, FL, 1983; 151-173.

22. Conrad ME, Umbreit JN, Moore EG et al. Mobilferrin, a homoloque of Ro/SS-A autoantigen and calreticulin. Blood 1991; 78:89a.

23. Fliegel L, Burns K, Wlasichuk K et al. Peripheral proteins of sarcoplasmic and endoplasmic reticulum. Biochem Cell Biol 1989; 67:696-702.

24. Mazzarella RA, Green M. ERp99, an abundant, conserved glycoprotein of the endoplasmic reticulum, is homologous to the 90-kDa heat shock protein (hsp90) and the 94-kDa glucose regulated protein (GRP94). J Biol Chem 1987; 262:8875-8883.

25. Mazzarella RA, Srinivasan M., Haugejorden SM et al. Erp72, an abundant luminal endoplasmic reticulum protein, contains three copies of the active site sequences of protein disulfide isomerase. J Biol Chem 1990; 265:1094-1101.

26. Michalak M, Milner RE. Calreticulin—a functional analogue of calsequestrin? Basic App Myol 1991; 1:121-128.

27. Unnasch TR, Gallin MY, Soboslay PT et al. Isolation and characterization of expression cDNA clones encoding antigens of *Onchocerca volvulus* infective larvae. J Clin Invest 1988; 82:262-269.

28. Bergeron JGM, Brenner MB, Thomas DY et al. Calnexin: a membrane-bound chaperone of the endoplasmic reticulum. TIBS 1994; 19:124-128.

29. Tjoelker LW, Seyfried CE, Eddy RL Jr et al. Human, mouse, and rat calnexin cDNA cloning: Identification of potential calcium binding motifs and gene localization to human chromosome 5. Biochemistry 1994; 33:3229-3236.

30. Malhotra R, Willis AD, Jensenius JC et al. Structure and homology of human C1q receptor (collectin receptor). Immunol 1993; 78:341-348.

31. Nigam SK, Goldberg AL, Ho S et al. A set of endoplasmic reticulum proteins possessing properties of molecular chaperones includes Ca^{2+}-binding proteins and members of the thioredoxin superfamily. J Biol Chem 1994; 269:1744-1749.

32. Neusfee WM, McCormick SJ, Clark RA. Calreticulin functions as a molecular chaperone in the biosynthesis of myeloperoxidase. J Biol Chem 1995; 270:4741-4747.

33. Liu N, Fine RE, Johnson RJ. Comparison of cDNA from bovine brain coding for two isoforms of calreticulin. Biochim Biophys Acta 1993; 1202:70-76.

34. Ohnishi M, Reithmeier RAF. Fragmentation of rabbit skeletal muscle calsequestrin: spectral and ion binding properties of the carboxyl-terminal region. Biochemistry 1987; 26:7458-7465.

35. Kennedy TE, Kuhl D, Barzilai A et al. Long-term sensitization training in *aplysia* leads to an increase in calreticulin, a major presynaptic calcium binding protein. Neuron 1992; 9:1013-1024.

36. Nakamura M, Moriya M, Baba T et al. An endoplasmic reticulum protein, calreticulin, is transported into the acrosome of rat sperm. Exp Cell Res 1993; 205:101-110.

37. Davies TW. *Schistosoma mansoi*: the structure and elemental composition of the pre-acetabullar penetration gland cell secretion in pre-emergent cercariae. Parasitology 1983; 87:55-60.

38. Khalife J, Liu JL, Pierce R et al. Characterization and localization of *Schistosoma mansoni* calreticulin Sm58. Parasitology 1994; 108:527-532.

39. Hawn TR, Tom TD, Strand M. Molecular expression of SmIrV1, a *Schistosoma mansoni* antigen with similarity to calnexin, calreticulin, and OvRal1. J Biol Chem 1993; 268:7692-7698.

40. Kretsinger RH, Moncrief ND, Goodman M et al. Homology of calcium modulated proteins: their evolutionary and functional relationships. In: Monrad M, Naylor WG, Kazda S, Schramm M, ed. The calcium channel, structure, function and implication. Springer-Verlag, 1988; 16-34.

41. Khanna NC, Takuda M, Waisman DM. Conformational changes induced by binding of divalent cations to calregulin. J Biol Chem 1986; 261:8883-8887.

42. Heilmann C, Spamer C, Leberer E et al. Human liver calreticulin. Characterization and Zn^{2+}-dependent interaction with phenyl-Sepharose. Biochem Biophys Res Commun 1993; 193:611-616.

43. Wada I, Rindress D, Cameron P et al. SSRα and associated calnexin are major calcium binding proteins of the endoplasmic reticulum membrane. J Biol Chem 1991; 266:19599-19610.

44. De Virgilio C, Bürckert N, Neuhaus J-M et al. CNE1, a *Saccharomyces cerevisiae* homologure of the genes encoding mammalian calnexin and calreticulin. Yeast 1993; 9:185-188.

45. Parlati F, Dominigues M, Bergeron JJM et al. *Saccharomyces cerevisiae* CNE1 encodes an endoplasmic reticulum (ER) membrane protein with sequence similarity to calnexin and calreticulin and functions as a constituent of the ER quality control apparatus. J Biol Chem 1995; 270:244-253.

46. Jannatipuor M, Rokeach LA. The *Schizosaccharomyces pombe* homologue of the chaperone calnexin is essential for viability. J Biol Chem 1995; 270:4845-4853.

CHAPTER 3

THE INTRACELLULAR DISTRIBUTION AND EXPRESSION OF CALRETICULIN

Michal Opas

THE LOCALIZATION OF CALRETICULIN TO THE ENDOPLASMIC/SARCOPLASMIC RETICULUM

Calreticulin is a 60-kDa Ca^{2+} binding protein that was originally identified in the sarcoplasmic reticulum of skeletal muscle (Chapter 1).[1] Despite this, its abundance in skeletal muscle is actually rather low,[2,3] and localization of the protein in differentiated skeletal muscle proved rather difficult. For this reason, at the outset of a collaborative study to determine the subcellular localization of calreticulin, we attempted to localize the protein in myoblasts (it had been detected in these cells in earlier biochemical studies).[4] While examining primary cultures of skeletal muscle it quickly became obvious that the cells which expressed calreticulin most abundantly were the fibroblasts that contaminated our muscle cultures. We decided, therefore, to screen a variety of cell types (using Western blotting) to determine the tissue distribution of calreticulin and we detected the protein in all cell types we examined.

The "typical" arrangement of anti-calreticulin labeling that we have seen is shown in Figure 3.1. Our localization studies, in several cell types, have shown that calreticulin co-distributes with the membrane system of the endoplasmic reticulum. Although we

---

found no evidence for the existence of the specialized, calsequestrin-rich Ca^{2+} storage vesicles, or calciosomes,[5] that have been described by others in several non-muscle cell types,[6,7] our results did not exclude the possibility that calreticulin may be sub-localized to specialized areas of the endoplasmic reticulum.

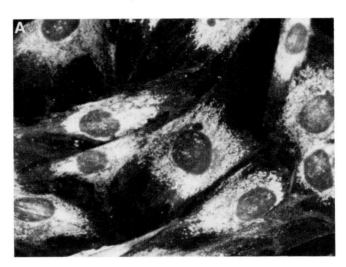

Fig. 3.1A

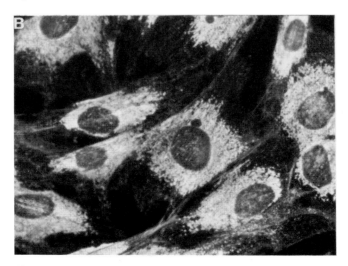

Fig. 3.1B

Fig. 3.1. Immunofluorescence microscopic localization of calreticulin in cells from a rat pigment epithelial cell line that were double labelled with specific antibodies against calreticulin and with TRITC-Con A. (B) shows the arrangement of the endoplasmic reticulum. (A) shows that calreticulin localizes predominantly to the endoplasmic reticulum-like intracellular network. The intranuclear localization of the calreticulin-like antigen(s) to groups of foci corresponding to nucleoli is quite apparent (see the text for further details).

To investigate the distribution of calreticulin with respect to structures associated with the endoplasmic reticulum, we quadruple-labelled L6 myoblasts.[8] The cells were initially stained with acridine orange to show ribosomes, and then restained with a fluorescent lipophilic probe, $DiOC_6$, to show the entire system of intracellular membranes. Finally the same cells were double-labeled with fluorescent-tagged concanavalin A, to show the arrangement of the endoplasmic reticulum, and with anti-calreticulin antibodies. We found an exact correspondence between the localization of calreticulin and the endoplasmic reticulum, and a high degree of correspondence between the distribution of calreticulin and ribosomes. Since the non-selective lipid staining was more extensive than the staining with anti-calreticulin we concluded that calreticulin may be confined to the rough endoplasmic reticulum.

Calreticulin is relatively abundant in cardiac muscle,[2,9] in contrast to skeletal muscle, allowing us to attempt to localize calreticulin within the cardiac myocyte. When embryonic cardiomyocytes are grown in cell culture they de-differentiate, develop stress fibres and look very much like fibroblasts. However, they then start to differentiate again, develop nascent myofibrils, and ultimately become beating myocytes filled with myofibrils. We studied the localization of calreticulin in these cells in order to determine whether the protein is present in the endoplasmic reticulum or whether it is associated with the myofibrils. Figure 3.2 shows that calreticulin in cardiac myocytes is not associated with myofibrils, and even seems to be excluded from the space occupied by the myofibrils. In contrast, calsequestrin is associated with the myofibrils in a typical striated pattern.

In other studies, we have immunoassayed plant tissues for calreticulin and have detected the protein in extracts from *Beta vulgaris, Tradescantia sp.*, and common grass. Interestingly, in sugar beet protoplasts that were attached to microscope slides via poly-L-lysine, fixed, permeabilized in Triton-containing buffer and stained for calreticulin, we detected the protein in the endoplasmic reticulum-like vesicular distribution that surrounds the large vacuole (unpublished).

The results of the above, and numerous additional, studies (carried out by ourselves[2,5,8,10,11] and by others[12-15]) have clearly shown that calreticulin is resident in the endoplasmic/sarcoplasmic reticulum. Furthermore, it has been shown recently that during mitosis and cell division the distribution of calreticulin closely follows that of the endoplasmic reticulum,[16] indicating that calreticulin is retained within the endoplasmic reticulum even during its most dynamic reorganization.

THE LOCALIZATION OF CALRETICULIN TO OTHER ORGANELLES

Calreticulin has been detected in organelles other than the endoplasmic reticulum. For example, the protein localizes specifically to the acrosome of sperm cells,[17] and to the cytotoxic granules in T cells (Chapter 9).[18] Further, it has been proposed that calreticulin may be localized to the cytoplasm.[19] Currently there is no direct evidence to support this suggestion, but we have recently detected calreticulin-like immunoreactivity in the cytoplasm of L cells, using anti-K-P-E-D-W-D synthetic peptide antibodies (unpublished observations).

Although not yet clearly identified, a calreticulin-like antigen has been detected in the nucleus of some cells.[8] Specifically, our anti-calreticulin antibody recognizes an antigen in the nuclei of several cell lines. Since the primary sequence of calreticulin contains

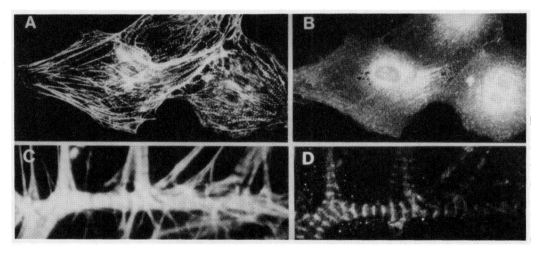

Fig. 3.2. The distribution of calreticulin (B), and calsequestrin (D), in de-differentiated chick embryo cardiac myocytes in vitro. Actin distribution in the same cells is shown in (A) and (C). Calreticulin is present in the endoplasmic reticulum of the cardiac myocytes, and is either distributed in a pattern not related to the myofibrillar organization or is excluded from the space occupied by myofibrils (B). The monoclonal anti-calsequestrin antibody used here shows that calsequestrin is found in a typical striated pattern in the cardiac myocytes (D). Please note the absence of nucleolar labelling with anti-calreticulin antibodies in these chick cells (see the text for further details).

a putative nuclear targeting signal it is not impossible that the protein might localize to the nucleus. However, in multiple localization studies we found that the intra-nuclear calreticulin-like antigen localized specifically to the nucleoli.[8,20] Furthermore, we have detected the intranuclear calreticulin-like antigen only in cells of rat origin (e.g. Fig. 3.1 but not Fig. 3.2). These observations lead us to suggest that the constitutive presence of calreticulin in the nucleus is an artifact.

THE EXPRESSION OF CALRETICULIN IN MUSCLE TISSUE

Since calreticulin is not abundantly expressed in differentiated muscle[2-4] we decided to investigate the regulation of its expression during muscle development, and to compare it with regulation of the expression of calsequestrin, the Ca^{2+} storage protein of striated muscle sarcoplasmic reticulum. To define the structural and temporal limits within which calreticulin and calsequestrin contribute to the phenotype of muscle tissue, we used the L6 myogenic cell line.[21] Although they do not develop into well-defined, striated myofibrils,[1] L6 myoblasts can be induced to differentiate into myotubes, in vitro.[22]

Calsequestrin was barely detectable, by Western blotting, in proliferating myoblasts, whereas its expression increased dramatically during differentiation. In cells which had been differentiating for several days, both unfused and fused, calsequestrin was present in a diffusely reticular, perinuclear and cytoplasmic arrangement. In contrast, calreticulin was detected, by immunoblotting, both before and throughout differentiation of the L6 cells. The level of neither calreticulin nor its message changed appreciably during L6 differentiation, and in both the L6 myoblasts and the myotubes calreticulin was localized to perinuclear areas.

Since L6 myotubes do not achieve full structural differentiation, we complemented these studies by localizing calreticulin and calsequestrin in fully differentiated muscle. We triple-labeled sections of adult rat skeletal muscle with anti-calreticulin and anti-calsequestrin antibodies, and with a DNA marker. While calsequestrin was present only in the sarcoplasmic reticulum, calreticulin was localized to perinuclear regions as well as to the sarcoplasmic reticulum. Thus both Ca^{2+} binding proteins are expressed in fully differentiated muscle, but with somewhat different distributions. Similar observations have been made in primary cultures of chick embryonic skeletal muscle.[23]

Calreticulin is present in the sarcoplasmic reticulum of muscle, but is also a major Ca^{2+} binding protein in the endoplasmic reticulum of non-muscle cells.[24] The expression and localization studies described above therefore support the suggestion that there are two separate Ca^{2+} storage pools in differentiated skeletal muscle, the endoplasmic reticulum and the sarcoplasmic reticulum. The sarcoplasmic reticulum is the Ca^{2+} pool which releases the Ca^{2+} required for contraction. The endoplasmic reticulum, on the other hand, may play a role in storage and release of the Ca^{2+} required for general cellular maintenance functions, including responses to extra-cellular signaling.[25]

A ROLE FOR CALRETICULIN IN CELL ADHESION?

Calreticulin binds Ca^{2+} with a high capacity ($B_{max} > 25$ moles of Ca^{2+}/mole of protein) and low affinity ($K_d = 250$ μM), and with a high affinity and low capacity ($K_d = 1$ μM, $B_{max} = 1$ mole of Ca^{2+}/mole of protein) (Chapter 2).[24,26] Because of its high binding capacity, calreticulin was proposed to be a Ca^{2+} storage protein in the lumen of the endoplasmic/sarcoplasmic reticulum (Chapter 5).[11] However, recent evidence indicates that calreticulin may have other role(s) to play in cellular function. In particular, calreticulin has been shown to modulate gene transcription regulated by the androgen and glucocorticoid receptors (Chapter 6).[27,28] These studies, and others, have led to the suggestion that calreticulin may be an important element in cell signaling.[19,29-31]

More recent evidence suggests that calreticulin might play some role in regulation of cell adhesion. In cell adhesion, the functions of both the cytoskeleton and cell surface receptors are regulated by Ca^{2+}, indicating that Ca^{2+} binding proteins likely play a role in these processes.[32] Currently, the mechanisms involved in regulation of cell adhesion, and of proper cytoskeleton function, are not fully elucidated. However, it has been shown that transient down-regulation of calreticulin affects adhesiveness of cells in culture,[33] and it has been suggested, therefore, that calreticulin may be involved in the regulation of cell adhesiveness.[33,34] In addition, our preliminary work shows profound effects of calreticulin over-expression upon adhesion and proliferation of L fibroblasts. Specifically, L fibroblasts that are over-expressing calreticulin flatten out, develop strong cell-substratum adhesions and, most surprisingly, establish epithelial-like cell–cell junctions.

Integrins, proteins which are involved in many endothelial cell functions, are heterodimers of α- and β- subunits that require Ca^{2+} for activity. At this writing, 16 α- and 8 β-integrin subunits have been described, and it is more than certain that this list will grow. The functional diversity of integrins occurs because each of the combinations of α- and β-subunits shows differing ligand specificity, and also because some integrins show a less-than-strict ligand selectivity, (e.g., $α_2β_1$ or $α_vβ_3$), especially when expressed on different cell types.

In an adhesive event, such as firm attachment of a leucocyte to endothelium or establishment of first contact with a substratum by a freshly plated cell in vitro, clustering and immobilization of integrins is crucial for adhesion-mediated cell signaling to occur,[35,37] possibly via tyrosine kinase activation.[38] More importantly, however, integrins must be activated, i.e. increase their affinity for ligands, in order for an adhesive event to occur.[39-43] Although ligand binding is associated with phosphorylation of the cytoplasmic domains of several integrins[44-50] a role for these phosphorylations in activation of integrins has not been established. It does appear, however, that a highly conserved amino acid sequence, K-x-G-F-F-K-R, found in the cytoplasmic domain of the α-subunits of integrins, is crucial for regulation of integrin affinity as its deletion locks integrins in a default, high affinity binding state.[31,51,52] Interestingly, calreticulin binds specifically to this highly conserved amino acid sequence.[34] The effects of calreticulin under/overexpression on cell adhesion, described above, may be mediated by interaction between calreticulin and the K-x-G-F-F-K-R amino acid sequence conserved in the cytoplasmic tails of α-integrins.[31,33,34,51]

ACKNOWLEDGMENTS

I would like to thank Ewa Dziak, Malgosia Szewczenko-Pawlikowski and Suzanne Tharin for their contribution to various aspects of research carried out in my laboratory as well as for just bearing with me. The continuous intellectual input and support of Dr. Marek Michalak (Department of Biochemistry, University of Alberta) is greatly appreciated. The mouse monoclonal antibody against skeletal muscle calsequestrin was a kind gift from

Dr. A. Jorgensen (Department of Anatomy and Cell Biology, University of Toronto). The rat pigment epithelial cell line was a generous gift of Dr. E. Rodriguez-Boulan (Department of Cell Biology and Anatomy, Cornell University). This work was supported by a grant from the Heart and Stroke Foundation of Ontario to M.O.

REFERENCES

1. Ostwald TJ, MacLennan DH. Isolation of a high affinity calcium binding protein from sarcoplasmic reticulum. J Biol Chem 1974; 249:974-9.
2. Fliegel L, Burns K, Opas M et al. The high-affinity calcium binding protein of sarcoplasmic reticulum. Tissue distribution, and homology with calregulin. Biochim Biophys Acta 1989; 982:1-8.
3. Tharin S, Dziak E, Michalak M et al. Widespread tissue distribution of rabbit calreticulin, a non-muscle functional analogue of calsequestrin. Cell Tissue Res 1992; 269:29-37.
4. Michalak M, MacLennan DH. Assembly of sarcoplasmic reticulum. Biosynthesis of the high affinity calcium binding protein in rat skeletal muscle cultures. J Biol Chem 1980; 255:1327-34.
5. Michalak M, Baksh S, Opas M. Identification and immunolocalization of calreticulin in pancreatic cells: no evidence for "calciosomes". Exp Cell Res 1991; 197:91-9.
6. Meldolesi J, Madeddu L, Pozzan T. Intracellular Ca^{2+} storage organelles in non-muscle cells: heterogeneity and functional assignment. Biochim Biophys Acta 1990; 1055:130-40.
7. Krause KH. Ca^{2+}-storage organelles. FEBS Lett 1991; 285:225-9.
8. Opas M, Dziak E, Fliegel L et al. Regulation of expression and intracellular distribution of calreticulin, a major calcium binding protein of nonmuscle cells. J Cell Physiol 1991; 149:160-71.
9. Wientzek M, Katz S. Isolation and characterization of purified sarcoplasmic reticulum membranes from isolated adult rat ventricular myocytes. J Mol Cell Cardiol 1991; 23:1149-63.
10. Fliegel L, Burns K, MacLennan DH et al. Molecular cloning of the high affinity calcium-binding protein (calreticulin) of skeletal muscle sarcoplasmic reticulum. J Biol Chem 1989; 264:21522-8.
11. Milner RE, Baksh S, Shemanko C et al. Calreticulin, and not calsequestrin, is the major calcium binding protein of smooth muscle sarcoplasmic reticulum and liver endoplasmic reticulum. J Biol Chem 1991; 266:7155-65.
12. Smith MJ, Koch GLE. Multiple zones in the sequence of calreticulin (CRP55, calregulin, HACBP), a major calcium binding ER/SR protein. EMBO J 1989; 8:3581-6.
13. Treves S, De Mattei M, Landfredi M et al. Calreticulin is a candidate for a calsequestrin-like function in Ca^{2+}-storage compartments (calciosomes) of liver and brain. Biochem J 1990; 271:473-80.

14. Krause K-H, Simmerman HKB, Jones LR et al. Sequence similarity of calreticulin with a Ca^{2+}-binding protein that co-purifies with an $Ins(1,4,5)P_3$-sensitive Ca^{2+} store in HL-60 cells. Biochem J 1990; 270:545-8.

15. Perrin D, Sönnichsen B, Söling H-D et al. Purkinje cells of rat and chicken cerebellum contain calreticulin (CaBP3). FEBS Lett 1991; 294:47-50.

16. Ioshii SO, Yoshida T, Imanaka-Yoshida K et al. Distribution of a Ca^{2+} storing site in PtK_2 cells during interphase and mitosis. An immunocytochemical study using an antibody against calreticulin. Eur J Cell Biol 1995; 66:82-93.

17. Nakamura M, Moriya M, Baba T et al. An endoplasmic reticulum protein, calreticulin, is transported into the acrosome of rat sperm. Exp Cell Res 1993; 205:101-10.

18. Dupuis M, Schaerer E, Krause KH et al. The calcium-binding protein calreticulin is a major constituent of lytic granules in cytolytic T lymphocytes. J Exp Med 1993; 177:1-7.

19. Burns K, Atkinson EA, Bleackley RC et al. Calreticulin: From Ca^{2+} binding to control of gene expression. TICB 1994; 4:152-4.

20. Opas M, Michalak M. Calcium storage in non-muscle tissues: is the retina special? Biochem Cell Biol 1992; 70:972-9.

21. Tharin S, Hamel PA, Conway E et al. Regulation of expression and distribution of calreticulin and calsequestrin during L6 skeletal muscle differentiation. J Cell Physiol 1995.[In Press]

22. Yaffe D. Retention of differentiation potentialities during prolonged cultivation of myogenic cells. Proc Natl Acad Sci USA 1968; 61:477-83.

23. Koyabu S, Imanaka-Yoshida K, Ioshii SO et al. Switching of the dominant calcium sequestering protein during skeletal muscle differentiation. Cell Motil Cytoskeleton 1994; 29:259-70.

24. Michalak M, Milner RE, Burns K et al. Calreticulin. Biochem J 1992; 285:681-92.

25. Berridge MJ. Inositol trisphosphate and calcium signalling. Nature 1993; 361:315-25.

26. Baksh S, Michalak M. Expression of calreticulin in *Escherichia coli* and identification of its Ca^{2+} binding domains. J Biol Chem 1991; 266:21458-65.

27. Burns K, Duggan B, Atkinson EA et al. Modulation of gene expression by calreticulin binding to the glucocorticoid receptor. Nature 1994; 367:476-80.

28. Dedhar S, Rennie PS, Shago M et al. Inhibition of nuclear hormone receptor activity by calreticulin. Nature 1994; 367:480-3.

29. Dedhar S. Novel functions for calreticulin: Interaction with integrins and modulation of gene expression. TIBS 1994; 19:269-71.

30. Nash PD, Opas M, Michalak M. Calreticulin: not just another calcium-binding protein. Mol Cell Biochem 1994; 135:71-8.

31. Williams MJ, Hughes PE, O'Toole TE et al. The inner world of

cell adhesion: integrin cytoplasmic domains. Trends Cell Biol 1994; 4:109-12.

32. Burridge K, Fath K, Kelly T et al. Focal adhesions: transmembrane junctions between the extracellular matrix and the cytoskeleton. Annu Rev Cell Biol 1988; 4:487-525.

33. Leung-Hagesteijn C-Y, Milankov K, Michalak M et al. Cell attachment to extracellular matrix substrates is inhibited upon downregulation of expression of calreticulin, an intracellular integrin α-subunit-binding protein. J Cell Sci 1994; 107:589-600.

34. Rojiani MV, Finlay BB, Gray V et al. In vitro interaction of a polypeptide homologous to human Ro/SS-A antigen (calreticulin) with a highly conserved amino acid sequence in the cytoplasmic domain of integrin subunits. Biochemistry 1991; 30:9859-66.

35. Schwartz MA, Lechene C, Ingber DE. Insoluble fibronectin activates the Na/H antiporter by clustering and immobilizing integrin $\alpha_5\beta_1$, independent of cell shape. Proc Natl Acad Sci USA 1991; 88:7849-53.

36. Lipp P, Niggli E. Ratiometric confocal Ca^{2+}-measurements with visible wavelength indicators in isolated cardiac myocytes. Cell Calcium 1993; 14:359-72.

37. McNamee HP, Ingber DE, Schwartz MA. Adhesion to fibronectin stimulates inositol lipid synthesis and enhances PDGF-induced inositol lipid breakdown. J Cell Biol 1993; 121:673-8.

38. Schaller MD, Parsons JT. Focal adhesion kinase: An integrin-linked protein tyrosine kinase. Trends Cell Biol 1993; 3:258-62.

39. Shimizu Y, van Seventer GA, Horgan KJ et al. Regulated expression and binding of three VLA (beta 1) integrin receptors on T cells. Nature 1990; 345:250-3.

40. Schweighoffer T, Shaw S. Adhesion cascades: Diversity through combinatorial strategies. Curr Opin Cell Biol 1992; 4:824-9.

41. Ginsberg MH, Du X, Plow EF. Inside-out integrin signalling. Curr Opin Cell Biol 1992; 4:766-71.

42. Du X, Plow EF, Frelinger AL, III et al. Ligands "activate" integrin $\alpha_{IIb}\beta_3$ (platelet GPIIb-IIIa). Cell 1991; 65:409-16.

43. Frelinger AL III, Du X, Plow EF et al. Monoclonal antibodies to ligand-occupied conformers of integrin $\alpha_{IIb}\beta_3$ (glycoprotein IIb-IIIa) alter receptor affinity, specificity, and function. J Biol Chem 1991; 266:17106-11.

44. Shaw LM, Messier JM, Mercurio AM. The activation dependent adhesion of macrophages to laminin involves cytoskeletal anchoring and phosphorylation of the $\alpha_6\beta_1$ integrin. J Cell Biol 1990; 110:2167-74.

45. Buyon JP, Slade SG, Reibman J et al. Constitutive and induced phosphorylation of the α and β chains of the CD11/CD18 leukocyte integrin family: Relationship to adhesion-dependent functions. J Immunol 1990; 144:191-7.

46. Haimovich B, Aneskievich BJ, Boettiger D. Cellular partitioning

of beta-1 integrins and their phosphorylated forms is altered after transformation by Rous sarcoma virus or treatment with cytochalasin D. Cell Regul 1991; 2:271-83.

47. Marcantonio EE, Guan JL, Trevithick JE et al. Mapping of the functional determinants of the integrin beta 1 cytoplasmic domain by site-directed mutagenesis. Cell Regul 1990; 1:597-604.

48. Freed E, Gailit J, Van der Geer P et al. A novel integrin beta subunit is associated with the vitronectin receptor alpha subunit (alpha v) in a human osteosarcoma cell line and is a substrate for protein kinase C. EMBO J 1989; 8:2955-65.

49. Aneskievich BJ, Haimovich B, Boettiger D. Phosphorylation of integrin in differentiating ts-Rous sarcoma virus-infected myogenic cells. Oncogene 1991; 6:1381-90.

50. Shaw LM, Mercurio AM. Regulation of $\alpha_6\beta_1$ integrin laminin receptor function by the cytoplasmic domain of the 6 subunit. J Cell Biol 1993; 123:1017-25.

51. O'Toole TE, Katagiri Y, Faull RJ et al. Integrin cytoplasmic domains mediate inside-out signal transduction. J Cell Biol 1994; 124:1047-59.

52. Ylänne J, Chen Y, O'Toole TE, et al. Distinct functions of integrin and subunit cytoplasmic domains in cell spreading and formation of focal adhesions. J Cell Biol 1993; 122:223-33.

THE ROLES OF CALNEXIN AND CALRETICULIN AS ENDOPLASMIC RETICULUM MOLECULAR CHAPERONES

**Frank Parlati, Richard Hemming, Wei-Jia Ou,
John J.M. Bergeron and David Y. Thomas**

INTRODUCTION

The endoplasmic reticulum is the entry point into the secretory pathway for the majority of soluble secreted proteins and membrane proteins (collectively termed secretory proteins). Within the endoplasmic reticulum secretory proteins have their signal peptide cleaved, they become extensively modified, they may associate with lipids, they become folded, they are N- and O-glycosylated, their disulfide bonds are formed and some are assembled into multimeric complexes.[1-3,8]

Correct folding of secretory proteins in the endoplasmic reticulum is essential for their transport to the subsequent compartments of the secretory pathway. The processes of protein translocation and folding in the endoplasmic reticulum are in close proximity and parts of a nascent translocating polypeptide chain can become N-glycosylated and start folding while their C-terminal region is still being translated. Folding of secretory proteins in the endoplasmic reticulum is mediated by molecular chaperones, and there

Calreticulin, edited by Marek Michalak. © 1996 R.G. Landes Company.

are also several endoplasmic reticulum proteins with enzymatic function which act as molecular chaperonins, including protein disulfide isomerase, and peptidyl prolyl *cis-trans* isomerase. N-linked glycosylation occurs on many secretory proteins and cells dedicate a large number of enzymes to this modification, but although glycosylation is a general feature of secretory proteins it is not always necessary for function. For example, glycosylation can be prevented and proteins are still secreted. Also the removal of oligosaccharides from proteins after secretion does not always alter their function.[5,6] Treatments which lead to the accumulation of unfolded proteins in the endoplasmic reticulum transcriptionally induce endoplasmic reticulum molecular chaperones.[5,7] Some misfolded or unassembled proteins are retained and proteolytically degraded either in the endoplasmic reticulum or in a later compartment of the secretory pathway.[8] This quality control function of the endoplasmic reticulum serves to prevent the secretion of incorrectly folded proteins or incompletely assembled cell surface complexes. In some cases it may serve as a control mechanism for secreted proteins, for example in the regulation of lipoprotein metabolism. An endoplasmic reticulum protein which has been shown to be a molecular chaperone for many secretory proteins is calnexin, and recent evidence is that the sequence related protein calreticulin also functions in the endoplasmic reticulum as a molecular chaperone.

THE FUNCTION OF CALNEXIN

The original cloning of calnexin occurred in a serendipitous fashion in a collaboration between our two groups. The initial impetus came from an observation that in isolated microsomes, endogenous protein kinases could phosphorylate a restricted subset of integral membrane proteins.[9] Calnexin was identified as a member of a complex of four integral membrane proteins. We named the protein of apparent 90-kDa molecular weight, calnexin, because of its similarity with calreticulin and our demonstration that it is one of the few endoplasmic reticulum membrane proteins which bind Ca^{2+}.[4] However, the function of calnexin remained enigmatic. The resolution of this dilemma came from the work of David Williams at the University of Toronto who had been investigating a protein, which he termed p88, which was associated with MHC I heavy chains during their maturation in the endoplasmic reticulum. Upon further analysis this protein proved to be identical with calnexin.[10] Other groups showed that calnexin was the protein associated with the assembly of a variety of cell surface oligomeric complexes, including major histocompatibility (MHC) class I and class II complexes, B cell and T cell receptors, integrin and nicotinic acetylcholine receptors.[11-17] It appeared that calnexin acts for these complexes as a molecular chaperone, that it is involved in the assembly of these complexes but is not a component of the finished complex. An unresolved question is the function of the original complex of endoplasmic reticulum proteins that we found in association with calnexin.[4]

We investigated whether calnexin was a general molecular chaperone for secretory glycoproteins or if it was restricted to assisting in the assembly of cell surface complexes. A key reagent for these studies was the development of anti-calnexin peptide polyclonal antibodies which could immunoprecipitate the native calnexin. We were able to immunoprecipitate calnexin from cell lysates under conditions which did not disrupt the interaction of calnexin with secretory proteins. To demonstrate the nature of calnexin as a molecular chaperone for many secretory proteins, we used HepG2 cells, which are derived from liver and which secrete a large number of well characterized secretory proteins for which antibodies are available.[18]

We set up a series of pulse-chase experiments after different treatments of HepG2, in which we were able to immunoprecipitate calnexin and associated proteins. Analysis of these immunoprecipitates by SDS polyacrylamide gel electrophoresis (SDS-PAGE) showed that at early times of the chase a large number of proteins could be detected in association with calnexin. This association was transient and proteins dissociated from calnexin with a measurable half-time of dissociation of the order of minutes. Using specific antibodies for secreted proteins and a sequential immunoprecipitation protocol we were able to identify some of the glycoproteins in association with calnexin. This protocol involved taking the primary immunoprecipitate made with the anti-calnexin antibody, dissociating the complex and then reprecipitating with a specific anti-glycoprotein antibody. In this way we were able to measure the association of glycoproteins with calnexin and their dissociation. The rates of dissociation from calnexin were significantly different for the various secretory glycoproteins tested. The

rank order of their half-times of association with calnexin was reflected in their relative rates of secretion from cells. That is to say,
the different rates of secretion of glycoproteins from cells is determined by the time of their association with calnexin. In support
of this conclusion, treatment of cells with the N-linked glycosylation inhibitor tunicamycin, which abrogates association of glycoproteins with calnexin (see below), results in their all being secreted from cells at a slow but uniform rate. Thus calnexin has a
major role and perhaps the major role in the secretion of many
glycoproteins.[18]

HOW DOES CALNEXIN RECOGNIZE ITS SUBSTRATES?

The HepG2 cell experimental system enabled us to establish
how calnexin recognizes its substrates. There are several lines of
evidence that calnexin binds to incompletely folded secretory proteins which are also N-glycosylated glycoproteins.

The unfolded state of the secretory glycoproteins in association with calnexin has been shown experimentally in several ways.
The state of folding of the secretory glycoprotein transferrin can
be followed by assessing the state of completeness of its disulfide
bonds by measuring its mobility on non-reducing polyacrylamide
gels. The forms of transferrin which were associated with calnexin
did not have all their disulfide bonds formed, but the other endoplasmic reticulum forms of transferrin that were not associated with
calnexin were folded.[18] Confirmation of this result comes from experiments in which we have coexpressed in the baculovirus-insect
cell system mammalian calnexin and the HIV-1 glycoprotein
gp120.[19,20] The state of folding of gp120 can be measured by its
association with the surface receptor CD4 which recognizes only
completely folded gp120. We have shown that gp120 which is
coimmunoprecipitated with calnexin cannot bind CD4 but that
the other endoplasmic reticulum forms of gp120 can bind CD4.
The interpretation of this result is that the forms of gp120 associated with calnexin are not in a conformation which can be recognized by CD4 and are thus incompletely folded, but that the other
form of gp120 in the endoplasmic reticulum can be recognized by
CD4 and is thus in the correct conformation. We have also ap-
proached this question by modifying the secretory glycoproteins.
Experimentally, the folding of proteins can be inhibited by the
incorporation of amino acid analogues such as the proline analogue

azetidine-2-carboxylic acid into proteins. Pulse chase and immu-noprecipitation studies with HepG2 cells which had been treated with azetidine-2-carboxylic acid showed that secretory glycopro-teins remained in association with calnexin for prolonged periods during the chase period.[18] Therefore calnexin retains incompletely folded proteins. Perhaps the best illustration that incompletely folded secretory glycoproteins proteins are bound to calnexin comes from studies of mutant secretory glycoproteins proteins. Mutant versions of proteins such as α_1-antitrypsin and the cystic fibrosis transmembrane regulator have been shown to have prolonged as-sociation with calnexin in the endoplasmic reticulum.[21,22] Calnexin thus forms part of an endoplasmic reticulum quality control appa-ratus which retains misfolded proteins in the endoplasmic reticulum and prevents their transport to later compartments. The consequence of this retention is that the retained proteins are proteolytically de-graded by an endoplasmic reticulum protease system.

From the study of the effects of the glycosylation inhibitor tunicamycin on HepG2 cells we established that calnexin requires proteins with which it associates to be N-glycosylated.[18] In addi-tion, we showed that the secretory glycoprotein α-fetoprotein as-sociates with calnexin, but that the closely sequence-related nonglycosylated protein serum albumin does not detectably associ-ate with calnexin.

Thus the evidence from pulse chase studies is that calnexin recognizes incompletely folded proteins which are N-glycosylated, it can also recognize subunits of unassembled oligomeric complexes, but it is not clear if the same mechanism of recognition is em-ployed for both classes of protein.

We have some information which identifies a region of calnexin which recognizes secretory glycoproteins. Expression of the HIV-1 gp120 with its natural signal sequence results in the retention of this glycoprotein in cells (Li et al, unpublished). Co-expression of the lumenal portion of mammalian calnexin results in its reten-tion in insect cells, presumably because of its association with the retained gp120 (Fig. 4.1).[20] Thus the region of calnexin respon-sible for the recognition of unfolded proteins lies within the lu-menal domain. We have also shown that the purified lumenal part of calnexin shares several properties with the full length protein, including protease resistance of a similar size core fragment in the presence of Ca^{2+}, the binding of ATP and oligomerization of the protein in the absence of Ca²⁺ or in the presence of added ATP.[20] Additional evidence for the function of this region also comes from the *Schizosaccharomyces pombe* calnexin *cnx1⁺* gene (Fig. 4.1). Deletion of *cnx1⁺* gives a lethal phenotype which is complemented by the expression of the lumenal domain of Cnx1p.[22,24] Although much of the deleted protein is detectable in the medium the cells are viable. What is not yet established is if the lethality of the *S. pombe cnx1* deletion mutants is due to the absence of the molecular chaperone function or to the absence of another function of calnexin.

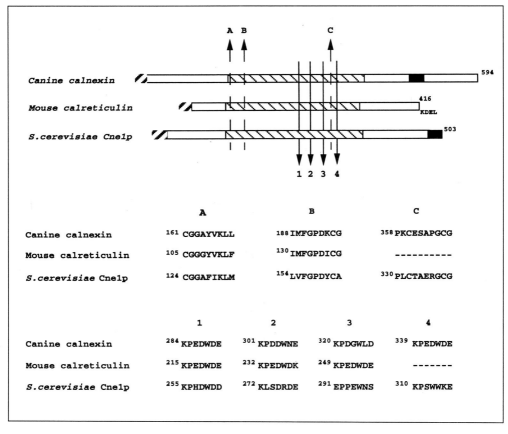

Fig. 4.1. Comparison of the conserved regions in mammalian calnexin and calreticulin and S. cerevisiae Cne1p. The signal sequence (▧) a highly conserved central domain (◳) and the transmembrane domain (■) are shown. Regions A, B and C code for conserved amino acids including cysteine residues. Regions 1, 2, 3 and 4 in the mammalian proteins, encode putative Ca²⁺ binding motifs (the corresponding amino acids in S. cerevisiae Cne1p are also denoted).

WHAT DOES CALNEXIN RECOGNIZE?

During the initial steps of N-glycosylation in eukaryotic cells the initial $Glc_3Man_9(GlcNAc)_2$ precursor, which is attached to the amide moiety of asparagine, is trimmed by the action of glucosidases I and II to $Man_9(GlcNAc)_2$ (Fig. 4.2).[6] There is then a remarkable reverse step in which the majority of newly synthesized proteins are reglucosylated by the enzyme UDP-glucose: glycoprotein glucosyltransferase (UGGT) which recognizes unfolded proteins (Fig. 4.2).[25] Observations on the glycosylation state of a mutant of VSV G protein (ts045) which is retained in the endoplasmic reticulum showed that it has a single glucose residue on N-linked oligosaccharides $(Glc_1Man_9(GlcNAc)_2)$. This glucose residue was added by the enzyme UGGT.[26] Next, calnexin was shown to form a stable complex with the ts045 mutant, and treatment of the cells with the glucosidase inhibitors castanospermine or 1-deoxynojirimycin abolished this association. On the basis of these in vivo results Helenius and coworkers proposed that calnexin recognizes the $Glc_1Man_9(GlcNAc)_2$ form of glycoproteins.[27]

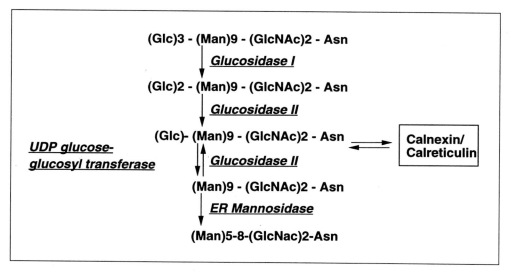

Fig. 4.2. Interaction between calnexin and N-linked oligosaccharide intermediates in the endoplasmic reticulum. Following the transfer of $(GlcNAc)_2$-$(Man)_9$-$(Glc)_3$ from the dolichol precursor to an asparagine residue on a secretory protein, two glucose residues are removed by the action of Glucosidases I & II. Proteins containing Asn-$(GlcNAc)_2$-$(Man)_9$-$(Glc)_1$ are bound by calnexin or by calreticulin. Incompletely folded proteins which possess an Asn-$(GlcNAc)_2$-$(Man)_9$ oligosaccharide are substrates for the enzyme UDP glucose: glycoprotein glucosyl transferase. This enzyme adds a single glucose residue to regenerate the Asn-$(GlcNAc)_2$-$(Man)_9$-$(Glc)_1$ intermediate which can then bind again to calnexin or calreticulin.

Direct support of this proposal has come from studies of the in vitro association of calnexin with isolated oligosaccharides and with monoglucosylated proteins. Of the $Glc_3Man_9(GlcNAc)_2$, $Glc_2Man_9(GlcNAc)_2$, and $Glc_1Man_9(GlcNAc)_2$ oligosaccharides only the latter binds to isolated calnexin, but this interaction is weak.[28] We have purified to homogeneity the lumenal domain of mammalian calnexin and cross linked it to magnetic beads. The N-glycosylated glycoproteins thyroglobulin and soy bean agglutinin do not bind strongly to calnexin. However, these proteins have some $Man_9(GlcNAc)_2$ oligosaccharides which are substrates for the enzyme UGGT when they are denatured. We purified UGGT and glucosylated these proteins in vitro with radioactive UDP-glucose. Using the calnexin binding assay we demonstrated high affinity and saturable binding of these $Glc_1Man_9(GlcNAc)_2$ proteins to calnexin. The binding is sensitive to Ca^{2+} chelators, but ATP had no effect. We were unable to efficiently compete the bound proteins with the monosaccharides which are commonly used to dissociate proteins from lectins, indicating that the oligosaccharide alone is not responsible for the binding that we observe. We then digested monoglucosylated thyroglobulin with different concentrations of proteinase K. With increased proteolysis of thyroglobulin the affinity for calnexin decreased (Ou et al, unpublished). One possible interpretation of this result is that the polypeptide links several $Glc_1Man_9(GlcNAc)_2$ residues, that there are several carbohydrate binding sites on calnexin, and that the effect we see is due to additivity of binding of several $Glc_1Man_9(GlcNAc)_2$ oligosaccharides. However, there are very few sites (<5%) which are receptive for monoglucosylation on thyroglobulin, and glycoproteins which have a single glycosylation site (e.g. soybean agglutinin and MHC I) bind to calnexin. Thus although the monoglucosylation of polypeptides is essential for their binding to calnexin, the presence of the peptide is essential for a high affinity interaction probably through peptide-peptide interactions. In support of this model, it has been shown in calnexin secretory protein coimmunoprecipitates that the glycan can be removed by digestion with endoglycosidase H, but that they remain associated. There are also reports of some nonglycosylated proteins associating with calnexin, again suggesting that polypeptides can bind calnexin.[8] A plausible model to account for these results is that monoglucosylated glycoproteins are initially recognized and bound by calnexin via their

$Glc_1Man_9(GlcNAc)_2$ moieties and that then the interaction of the polypeptide with calnexin occurs to give a higher affinity binding. An implication of these results is that dissociation of proteins from calnexin does not occur because of the trimming of the oligosaccharide by for example glucosidase II, but must occur by a different mechanism. One strong possibility is that the calnexin-polypeptide interaction is sensitive to secondary structure and that the state of folding determines the release of proteins from calnexin.

CALNEXIN AND CALRETICULIN COMPARED

Calnexin and calreticulin occur together in many eukaryotic organisms. There are several regions of shared amino acid motifs and this sequence similarity led us initially to examine the Ca^{2+} binding properties of calnexin, as calreticulin had been shown to be a Ca^{2+}-binding protein. The gene (*CNE1*) identified as calnexin in the yeast *Saccharomyces cerevisiae* is interesting in that it is the most divergent of the calnexin-calreticulin family. The overall sequence identity of Cne1p with mammalian calnexin is 24% and with mammalian calreticulin is 21%; thus it could be the homolgue of either protein. Although we have shown that like calnexin it is an integral endoplasmic reticulum membrane protein, it does not have a cytoplasmic domain as do all other calnexins. Calreticulin has been found to be involved in a variety of processes and pathologies (see other chapters in this volume).[29] There is a considerable sequence similarity between calnexin and calreticulin and they share a similar cellular location (Fig. 4.1)(Chapter 3) implying that they may have a similar function in the endoplasmic reticulum, namely as molecular chaperones, and function together as part of the endoplasmic reticulum quality control apparatus. Indeed, a good illustration of the direct role of calnexin in endoplasmic reticulum quality control is that deletion of the *S. cerevisiae CNE1* gene allows the secretion of mutant proteins from the cell. An indication that calreticulin might act as a molecular chaperone came from the demonstration that, along with many known endoplasmic reticulum molecular chaperones, it could bind to a column of denatured proteins.[32]

More direct evidence for this function came recently from antibodies which can efficiently immunoprecipitate calreticulin.[30] Using these antibodies, the lysosomal heme containing glycoprotein myeloperoxidase was shown to associate for prolonged periods with calreticulin. This result strongly suggested that calreticulin acts as a molecular chaperone for this protein. We used these antibodies to immunoprecipitate from pulse labeled HepG2 cells calreticulin in association with secretory glycoproteins. We have shown that, as with calnexin, this association of secretory proteins with calreticulin is transient (Hemming et al, unpublished). There seem to be many proteins which interact with calnexin and with calreticulin. The rate of dissociation of proteins from calreticulin is about the same as their as their rate of dissociation from calnexin. However, the strength of the signal of the interaction of proteins with calreticulin is about 10% of the signal observed for the same protein with calnexin. The association is inhibited by tunicamycin, showing that the associated proteins are glycoproteins and that they require glycosylation for the interaction. That lower amounts of secretory proteins associate with calreticulin with the same kinetics that they associate with calnexin (a less abundant protein) is an apparently paradoxical result.

We tested whether purified calreticulin could bind glycoproteins in vitro. We used the same assay that we used for calnexin binding with secretory glycoproteins. As with calnexin, calreticulin can bind glycoproteins which have the $Glc_1Man_9(GlcNAc)_2$ form of N-linked oligosaccharide (Ou et al, unpublished). However, in competition experiments calreticulin has 8-10 fold less affinity for these proteins. This latter result is in agreement with the observation of the weak association of calreticulin and glycoproteins in vivo.

In a direct test of the equivalence of the function of calnexin and calreticulin, Ikuo Wada and co-workers made recombinants of residues 1-340 of calreticulin (the lumenal domain) with residues 459-573 of calnexin (including the membrane spanning domain and the cytoplasmic domain, Fig. 4.1).[31] They incorporated an antibody tag into their constructions which would allow the proteins to be immunoprecipitated and distinguished from endogenous calnexin and calreticulin. Expressing these constructions in HepG2 cells allowed them to make a direct comparison with endogenous calnexin and calreticulin in these cells. They were able to show that the membrane attached form of calreticulin binds secretory proteins. Although a direct quantitation was not made, the membrane attached form of calreticulin seems to bind secretory proteins with a higher affinity than lumenal calreticulin.

Thus it appears that cells have two similar proteins in the same cellular location which apparently have similar functions. However, this coexistence is not obligatory, as an intensive search of the genome of the yeasts *Saccharomyces cerevisiae* and *Schizosaccharomyces pombe* has only revealed the presence of the calnexin related genes and a calreticulin homologue has not been found.[23,24] In addition the results from complementation of the *S. pombe cnx1* gene disruption has shown that the lethality can be complemented by a soluble (and eventually secreted) form of the Cnx1+ protein. This indicates that the membrane location of calnexin is not essential for its function and in this case it is acting like calreticulin in the lumen of the endoplasmic reticulum.

THE CURRENT MODEL

The current model of calnexin and calreticulin function places them both as molecular chaperones and members of the endoplasmic reticulum quality control apparatus. Secretory glycoproteins enter the endoplasmic reticulum and become N-glycosylated by the action of oligosaccharyl transferase, the glucose residues are trimmed by the successive action of glucosidase I, which removes the terminal glucose residue, and then glucosidase II, which removes the second and third glucose residues. It is not clear if there is an interaction of this monoglucosylated form of glycoproteins with calreticulin and calnexin, or if it is only the forms which have had the glucose residue re-added by UGGT which associate. Presumably for large glycoproteins it is possible that a single secretory glycoprotein molecule can simultaneously interact with several components of the import and chaperone machinery. UGGT recognizes unfolded proteins, particularly unfolded regions and reglucosylates them and they rebind calnexin or calreticulin. At present the evidence is that the release of proteins from calnexin is not mediated by removal of the oligosaccharide but possibly occurs after folding of the polypeptide by molecular chaperonins of the endoplasmic reticulum such as protein disulfide isomerase and peptidyl prolyl *cis-trans* isomerase.

It is not clear if calreticulin associates with glycoproteins after they have associated with calnexin or if they act simultaneously. However, there is clearly a weaker association of glycoproteins with calreticulin than with calnexin, even though the former is about ten times more abundant in the endoplasmic reticulum than the latter and the overall time of the association of glycoproteins with them is very similar. One model which could account for these findings is that there is a rapid exchange of glycoproteins between calnexin and calreticulin with more time being spent in association with the former than the latter. This would account for the overall rates of dissociation of secretory glycoproteins from calnexin and calreticulin being approximately the same. A clue to a different function for calnexin and calreticulin may come from their membrane and lumenal locations. Most molecular chaperones in the endoplasmic reticulum are lumenal proteins and there may be a role for calreticulin as opposed to calnexin in ensuring that glycoproteins encounter these proteins.

The finding that calnexin and calreticulin interact with a specific oligosaccharide motif on secretory proteins in order to retain them while they are being folded, suggests that oligosaccharide modifictions may be used may be used for other functions. It is already known that the mannose-6 phosphate modification is used as a lysosomal sorting determinant by a receptor in the *trans*-Golgi network.[33] And recently ERGIC-53, a membrane protein in the intermediate compartment, has been shown to be identical to a previously identified mannose binding protein.[34,35] It is possible that eukaryotic cells use oligosaccharide modifications on secretory proteins to sort and verify the status of glycoproteins at many steps in the secretory pathway and that many new oligosaccharide binding proteins will be found.

ACKNOWLEDGMENTS

The results from the authors' (JJMB and DYT) laboratories were supported by grants from the Medical Research Council of Canada.

REFERENCES

1. Gething MJ, Sambrook J. Protein folding in the cell. Nature 1992; 355:33-45.
2. Hurtley S, Helenius A. Protein oligomerization in the endoplasmic reticulum. Annu Rev Cell Biol 1989; 5:277-307.
3. Pelham HRB. Control of protein exit from the endoplasmic reticulum. Annu Rev Cell Biol 1989; 5:1-23.
4. Wada I, Rindress D, Cameron P et al. SSRα and associated calnexin are major calcium binding proteins of the endoplasmic reticulum membrane. J Biol Chem 1991; 266:19599-19610.

5. Bergeron JJM, Wada I, Thomas DY. Calnexin. In: Guidebook to the Secretory Pathway. Rothblatt J, Novick P, Stevens T, eds. Sambrook and Tooze publication at the Oxford University Press Inc: New York NY, 1994.

6. Elbein AD. Glycosidase inhibitors: inhibitors of N-linked oligosaccharide processing. FASEB J 1991; 5:3055-3063.

7. Klausner RD, Lippincott-Schwartz J, Bonifacino JS. The T cell antigen receptor: insights into organelle biology. Annu Rev Cell Biol 1990; 6:403-431.

8. Bergeron JJM, Brenner MB, Thomas DY et al. Calnexin: A membrane-bound chaperone of the endoplasmic reticulum. TIBS 1994; 19:124-128.

9. Rindress D, Lei X, Ahluwalia JPS et al. Organelle-specific phosphorylation: Identification of unique membrane phosphoproteins of the endoplasmic reticulum and endosomal apparatus. J Biol Chem 1993; 268:5139-5147.

10. Williams DB. Calnexin: a molecular chaperone with a taste for carbohydrate. Biochem Cell Biol 1995; 73: in press

11. Degen E, Williams DB. Participation of a novel 88 kDa protein in the biogenesis of murine class I histocompatibility molecules. J Cell Biol 1991; 112:1099-1115.

12. Hochstenbach F, David V, Watkins S et al. Endoplasmic reticulum resident protein of 90 kilodaltons associates with the T- and B-cell antigen receptors and major histocompatibility complex antigens during their assembly. Proc Natl Acad Sci USA 1992; 89:4734-4738.

13. Jackson MR, Cohen-Doyle MF, Peterson PA et al. Regulation of MHC class I transport by the molecular chaperone, calnexin (p88, IP90). Science 1994; 263:384-387.

14. Anderson KS, Cresswell P. A role for calnexin (IP90) in the assembly of class II MHC molecules. EMBO J 1994; 13:675-682.

15. David V, Hochstenbach F, Rajagopalan S et al. Interaction with newly synthesized and retained proteins in the endoplasmic reticulum suggests a chaperone function for human integral membrane protein IP90 (calnexin). J Biol Chem 1993; 268:9585-9592.

16. Lenter M, Vestweber D. The integrin chains β_1 and α_6 associate with the chaperone calnexin prior to integrin assembly. J Biol Chem 1994; 269:12263-12268.

17. Gelman MS, Chang W, Thomas DY et al. Role of the endoplasmic reticulum chaperone calnexin in subunit folding and assembly of nicotinic acetylcholine receptors. J Biol Chem 1995; 270: in press.

18. Ou W-J, Cameron P, Thomas DY et al. Association of folding intermediates of glycoproteins with calnexin during protein maturation. Nature 1993; 364:771-776.

19. Li Y, Lo L, Thomas DY, Kang CY. Positively charged amino acids on the signal sequence of human immunodeficiency virus gp120 control post-translational processing and secretion. Virology 1994; 204:266-278.

20. Ou WJ, Bergeron JJM, Li Y et al. Conformational changes in calnexin induced by Ca^{2+} and ATP. J Biol Chem 1995; 270: in press.

21. Le A, Steiner JL, Ferrell GA et al. Association between calnexin and a secretion-incompetent variant of human α_1-antitrypsin. J Biol Chem 1994; 269:7514-7519.

22. Pind S, Riordan J, Williams DB. Participation of the ER chaperone calnexin (p88, IP90) in the biogenesis of CFTR. J Biol Chem 1994; 269:12784-12788.

23. Parlati F, Dominguez M, Bergeron JJM et al. *Saccharomyces cerevisiae* CNE1, encodes an ER membrane protein with sequence similarity to calnexin and calreticulin and functions as a constituent of the ER quality control apparatus. J Biol Chem 1995; 270:244-253.

24. Parlati F, Dignard D, Bergeron JJM et al. *Schizosaccharomyces pombe* cnx1+ encodes the mammalian calnexin homologue that is an essential gene, heat shock inducible gene. EMBO J 1995; in press.

25. Trombetta SE, Parodi A. Purification to apparent homogeneity and partial characterization of rat liver UDP-glucose:glycoprotein glucosyltransferase. J Biol Chem 1992; 267:9236-9240.

26. Suh P, Bergmann JE, Gabal CA. Selective retention of monoglucosylated high mannose oligosaccharides by a class of mutant vesicular stomatitis virus G proteins. J Cell Biol 1989; 108:811-819.

27. Hebert DN, Foellmer B, Helenius A. Glucose trimming and reglucosylation determine glycoprotein association with calnexin in the endoplasmic reticulum. Cell 1995; 81:425-433.

28. Ware F, Vassilakos A, Peterson PA et al. The molecular chaperone calnexin binds $Glc_1Man_9GlcNAc_2$ oligosaccharide as an initial step in recognizing unfolded glycoproteins. J Biol Chem 1995; 270:4697-4704.

29. Nash PD, Opas M, Michalak M. Calreticulin: not just another calcium-binding protein. Mol Cell Biochem 1994; 135:71-78.

30. Nauseef WM, McCormick SJ, Clark RA. Calreticulin functions as a molecular chaperone in the biosynthesis of myeloperoxidase. J Biol Chem 1995; 270:4741-4747.

31. Wada I, Imai S, Kai M et al. Chaperone function of calreticulin when expressed in the endoplasmic reticulum as the membrane-anchored and soluble forms. J Biol Chem 1995; 270:20298-20304.

32. Nigam SK, Goldberg AL, Ho S et al. A set of endoplasmic reticulum proteins possessing properties of molecular chaperones includes Ca^{2+}-binding proteins and members of the thioredoxin superfamily. J Biol Chem 1994; 269:1744-1749.

33. Kornfeld S, Mellman I. The biogenesis of lysosomes. Annu Rev Cell Biol 1989; 5:483-525.
34. Arar C, Carpentier V, Le Caer J-P et al. ERGIC-53, a membrane protein of the enoplasmic reticulum-Golgi intermediate compartment, is identical to MR60, an intracellular mannose specific lectin of myelomonocytotic cells. J Biol Chem 1995; 270:3551-3553.
35. Fiedler K, Simons K. The role of N-glycans in the secretory pathway. Cell 1995; 81:309-312.

CHAPTER 5

CALRETICULIN AND CA²⁺ STORAGE

Karl-Heinz Krause

INTRODUCTION

CA²⁺ STORES

Ca^{2+} "stores" are intra-cellular compartments that are characterized by their high intra-luminal Ca^{2+} content, and by their participation in the regulation of cytosolic free Ca^{2+} concentration ($[Ca^{2+}]_c$) through rapid Ca^{2+} accumulation and release*. These Ca^{2+} stores, which are thought to reside either within the entire endoplasmic reticulum, within the rough endoplasmic reticulum, or within smooth-surfaced endoplasmic reticulum-subcompartments (for review see refs. 1-6) play a crucial role in stimulus response coupling. In resting cells, Ca^{2+} stores contain high concentrations of Ca^{2+}. During cellular activation this stored Ca^{2+} is released into the cytosol. $[Ca^{2+}]_c$ is around 100 nM in resting cells, but may increase to micromolar levels as Ca^{2+} is released. The release of Ca^{2+} from intracellular stores occurs through two families of Ca^{2+} release channels ($Ins(1,4,5)P_3$ receptors and ryanodine receptors).

There are other intracellular compartments that have a high intra-luminal Ca^{2+} content. Strictly speaking, all organelles that contain high intra-luminal Ca^{2+} concentrations may be called Ca^{2+} stores.[6] However, throughout this review we use the term Ca^{2+} stores to refer only to agonist-sensitive, rapidly exchangeable Ca^{2+} stores.

Calreticulin, edited by Marek Michalak. © 1996 R.G. Landes Company.

Ca²⁺ uptake into intracellular Ca²⁺ stores is energy-dependent and occurs through a family of Ca²⁺-ATPases (Sarco-Endoplasmic Reticulum Ca²⁺-ATPases=SERCA).

Intracellular Ca²⁺ stores, by definition, must store large amounts of Ca²⁺ within a restricted fraction of the cellular volume. For this reason, it is widely assumed that Ca²⁺ stores contain intra-luminal Ca²⁺ buffers to allow the accumulation of large amounts of Ca²⁺ without an excessive increase in the intra-luminal free Ca²⁺ concentration ($[Ca^{2+}]_s$). This buffering might be carried out by non-protein Ca²⁺ buffers (i.e. inorganic phosphate or various organic acids) and/or by Ca²⁺ binding proteins (i.e. Ca²⁺ storage proteins).

CALRETICULIN

The protein that is thought to make the most significant contribution to Ca²⁺ storage in muscle sarcoplasmic reticulum is calsequestrin.[7,8] Attempts were made, consequently, to locate calsequestrin in non-muscle cells, but it rapidly became clear that—with very few exceptions[9]—non-muscle cells do not contain calsequestrin.[10] However, when searching non-muscle cells for possible Ca²⁺ storage proteins, using non-specific screening procedures (⁴⁵Ca²⁺ overlay and Stains-all staining), several groups detected an abundant Ca²⁺ binding protein with an apparent molecular weight of approximately 60-kDa. Several different names were given to this protein, including CRP55,[11] calsequestrin-like protein,[12-14] and CaBP3.[15] Once the primary sequence of the protein had been deduced by cDNA cloning,[16,17] the name calreticulin (calcium binding protein of the sarco/endoplasmic reticulum) was agreed upon (Chapter 1). The primary sequence of calreticulin shows a highly acidic C-terminal domain, which is analogous, but not homologous, to that of calsequestrin. The protein has also been referred to as "a non-muscle functional analogue of calsequestrin".[18] By expressing different domains of calreticulin in *E. coli,* it was shown that this acidic C-domain is the portion of the molecule responsible for the protein's high capacity, low affinity Ca²⁺ binding (Chapter 2).[19]

While circumstantial evidence suggests a role for calreticulin in Ca²⁺ storage, it has been extremely difficult to provide scientific proof for this hypothesis. Indeed, to date, the question of whether or not calreticulin plays a relevant role in cellular Ca²⁺ storage remains open. The aim of this chapter is to review current knowledge of both quantitative and qualitative aspects of intra-luminal Ca^{2+} storage within intracellular Ca^{2+} stores. We will then summarize the evidence that indicates whether or not calreticulin might play a role as a Ca^{2+} storage protein in non-muscle cells.

WHAT IS THE TOTAL CA²⁺ CONCENTRATION WITHIN INTRACELLULAR CA²⁺ STORES?

One may obtain estimates of the total concentration of Ca^{2+} ($[Ca^{2+}]_{st}$) within intracellular Ca^{2+} stores from the following measurements: i) the amplitude of elevations in $[Ca^{2+}]_c$, ii) $^{45}Ca^{2+}$ release from intact cells and iii) electron probe X-ray microanalysis.

THE AMPLITUDE OF ELEVATIONS IN $[CA^{2+}]_C$

Using Ca^{2+}-sensitive fluorescent dyes, one can measure the amplitude of stimulated increases in $[Ca^{2+}]_c$. If these measurements are made in a Ca^{2+}-free medium, they reflect increases that are due to Ca^{2+} release from intracellular stores. Under these conditions, then, the maximal increases in $[Ca^{2+}]_c$ observed allow us to obtain a minimum estimate of the total Ca^{2+} concentration within intracellular Ca^{2+} stores. To make this calculation we need to estimate the i) cytosolic buffering capacity and ii) the relative Ca^{2+} store volume (Ca^{2+} store volume /total cellular volume) of a cell. Assuming a relative Ca^{2+} store volume of 0.02 (see also Fig. 5.1), and an average cytosolic Ca^{2+} binding capacity of 75 (i.e. 75 Ca^{2+} bound for 1 Ca^{2+} free[20] *), the $[Ca^{2+}]_{st}$ should be at least 3750-fold (i.e. cytosolic Ca^{2+} binding capacity/relative Ca^{2+} store volume) higher than the maximal cytosolic Ca^{2+} concentration that can be obtained through Ca^{2+} release. Since the maximal increases in $[Ca^{2+}]_c$ resulting from to Ca^{2+} release may exceed 1 µM in many cells types, $[Ca^{2+}]_{st}$ could be >3.75 mM. Note that these minimum estimates likely underestimate $[Ca^{2+}]_{st}$, because they assume i) a complete release of all stored Ca^{2+}, and ii) no relevant activation of Ca^{2+} pumps.

$^{45}CA^{2+}$ RELEASE FROM INTACT CELLS

A second method of estimating $[Ca^{2+}]_{st}$ involves measuring the amount of Ca^{2+} that can be released, after equilibrium incubation of cells with $^{45}Ca^{2+}$, by i) $Ins(1,4,5)P_3$-generating agonists or

---

* In the study to which we referred[20] the cytosolic buffering capacity was found to be constant, from the nanomolar to the low micromolar range.

ii) inhibitors of SERCA-type Ca^{2+}-ATPases. The calculations performed here are based on the results of a study conducted with the neuroblastoma cell line PC12.[21] A concentration of 0.2 mmole Ca^{2+}/liter of cell water was found. In these cells, again assuming a relative Ca^{2+} store volume of 0.02, $[Ca^{2+}]_{st}$ would be 10 mM.

The estimates made above both depend on the assumed relative Ca^{2+} store volume. However, no reliable measurements of relative Ca^{2+} store volume are available. Figure 5.1 shows the dependence of calculated $[Ca^{2+}]_{st}$ on the assumed relative Ca^{2+} store volume. Clearly, it is impossible to give precise numbers for $[Ca^{2+}]_{st}$ with our present knowledge. However, it is likely that $[Ca^{2+}]_{st}$ is very high compared with $[Ca^{2+}]_c$, perhaps above 10 mM. Previous reviews in the field have estimated $[Ca^{2+}]_{st}$ at between 5 and 50 mM.[2,22]

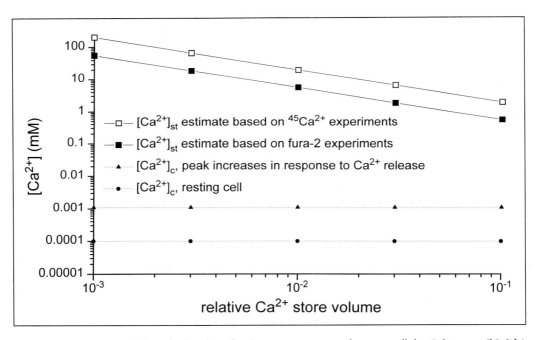

Fig. 5.1. Dependence of the calculated total Ca^{2+} concentration within intracellular Ca^{2+} stores ($[Ca^{2+}]_{st}$), on the assumed relative Ca^{2+} store volume. The relative Ca^{2+} store volume is defined as the ratio between the Ca^{2+} store volume and the total cellular volume. $[Ca^{2+}]_{st}$ estimations are based on fura-2 measurements. Calculations are based on a cell with a cytosolic Ca^{2+} binding capacity of 75[20] (i.e. 75 Ca^{2+} bound for 1 Ca^{2+} free) and a maximal $[Ca^{2+}]_c$ increase resulting from Ca^{2+} release of 1 μM. $[Ca^{2+}]_{st}$ is then ($[Ca^{2+}]_c$ increase x cytosolic buffering capacity)/ relative store volume. $[Ca^{2+}]_{st}$ estimations based on $^{45}Ca^{2+}$ measurements. Calculations are based on a cell with a Ca^{2+} store content of 0.2 mmole Ca^{2+}/liter of cell water.[21] $[Ca^{2+}]_{st}$ is then a direct function of the ratio of store volume/cell volume and can be calculated as Ca^{2+} store content per liter of cell water / relative store volume. To put the numbers into perspective, $[Ca^{2+}]_c$ values in resting cells and $[Ca^{2+}]_c$ peak increases in response to Ca^{2+} release are shown.

ELECTRON PROBE X-RAY MICROANALYSIS

This technique can be used to measure absolute ion concentrations within freeze-dried sections. The results obtained with this technique suggest that the Ca^{2+} content in endoplasmic reticulum-rich regions is between 5 and 50 mmol/kg dry weight (for example see refs. 23, 24). However, because these studies are done with freeze-dried material, it is difficult to convert the numbers to allow an estimate of the molar Ca^{2+} concentrations within Ca^{2+} stores.

WHAT ARE THE INTRA-LUMINAL BUFFERS OF INTRACELLULAR CA²⁺ STORES?

NON-PROTEIN CA²⁺ BUFFERS WITHIN INTRACELLULAR CA²⁺ STORES

The most likely relevant non-protein Ca^{2+} buffer within intracellular Ca^{2+} stores is inorganic phosphate (P_i). P_i is found in the cytosol of cells in low millimolar concentrations, appears to be able to permeate intracellular Ca^{2+} stores (as judged by studies in homogenized or permeabilized cells[25,26]) and forms a complex with Ca^{2+} that does not precipitate in Ca^{2+} concentrations of up to 50 mM.[25] However, owing to a relatively low association constant ($30 M^{-1}$),[25] a high intra-luminal concentration of P_i would be necessary to provide physiologically relevant Ca^{2+} buffering within the Ca^{2+} stores (Fig. 5.2A). Other candidates for non-protein Ca^{2+} buffers, within intracellular Ca^{2+} stores, are Ca^{2+}-complexing organic acids. Oxalate is widely used in studies of Ca^{2+} uptake by intracellular stores (for example see refs. 27, 28) and might act as an intra-luminal Ca^{2+} buffer. Other candidate organic acids include citrate, aspartate, and glutamate, all of which show low affinity Ca^{2+} binding. However, it is not known whether, under physiological conditions, there are relevant concentrations of these compounds within the lumen of intracellular Ca^{2+} stores.

CA²⁺ BINDING PROTEINS WITHIN INTRACELLULAR CA²⁺ STORES

A number of proteins that bind Ca^{2+} with low to intermediate affinity are situated within the lumen of the endoplasmic reticulum and might, therefore, contribute to Ca^{2+} storage. Besides calreticulin, such proteins include protein disulfide isomerase (PDI), BiP, Grp94 and others (for review see ref. 10). These intra-luminal Ca^{2+} binding proteins are referred to as "reticuloplasm" by some authors and their bulk Ca^{2+} binding properties include a low affinity

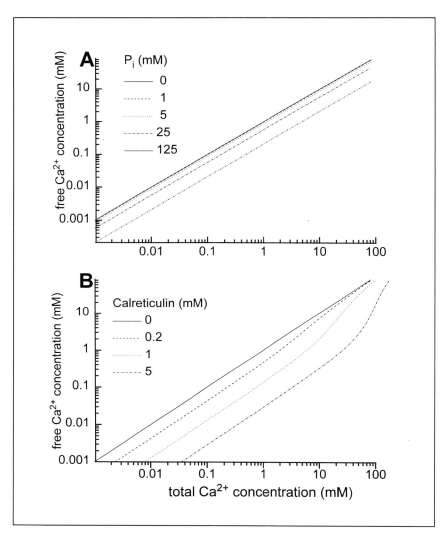

*Fig. 5.2. Relationship between [Ca²⁺]ₛₜ and [Ca²⁺]ₛ in phosphate-buffered, and calreticulin-buffered, systems. The relationship between [Ca²⁺]ₛₜ and [Ca²⁺]ₛ was calculated for different phosphate concentrations (panel **A**), and different calreticulin concentrations (panel **B**). A Kd for calcium phosphate of 33 mM[25] was used for the calculations. Ca²⁺ binding to calreticulin was calculated on the basis of 20 low affinity Ca²⁺ binding sites (Kd 1 mM), and 1 high affinity Ca²⁺ binding site (Kd 1 μM).[35] For phosphate, a constant free concentration was assumed (since the cytosol presumably acts as a very large reservoir). In contrast, for calreticulin, a constant total concentration was assumed. This explains the fact that the relationship between [Ca²⁺]ₛₜ and [Ca²⁺]ₛ is linear for phosphate, but sigmoidal for calreticulin.*

(K_d ~1 mM) with a capacity of 300 nmoles Ca^{2+}/mg endoplasmic reticulum protein.[11] As calreticulin is one of the most abundant of these proteins, and has the highest number of Ca^{2+} binding sites, it is likely to account for an important part of the observed "bulk" Ca^{2+}-binding capacity (for example see refs. 29 and 30). Figure 5.2B shows the impact of three different intra-luminal calreticulin concentrations on the relationship between the total Ca^{2+} concentration, $[Ca^{2+}]_{st}$, and the free Ca^{2+} concentration, $[Ca^{2+}]_s$, (assuming that calreticulin is the exclusive Ca^{2+} buffer in the system).

WHAT IS THE FREE CA²⁺ CONCENTRATION WITHIN INTRACELLULAR CA²⁺ STORES?

Since there are numerous intra-luminal Ca^{2+} buffers, the free Ca^{2+} concentration within intracellular Ca^{2+} stores ($[Ca^{2+}]_s$), is likely not identical with the total Ca^{2+} concentration ($[Ca^{2+}]_{st}$). For several decades researchers have been interested in measuring this free Ca^{2+} concentration within intracellular Ca^{2+} stores. So far, three different approaches have been used to obtain estimates of $[Ca^{2+}]_s$.

OXALATE AND PHOSPHATE ENHANCEMENT OF CA²⁺ UPTAKE

An enhancement of Ca^{2+} uptake, in homogenates and permeabilized cells of both muscle and non-muscle tissues, results from the addition of oxalate or phosphate. As both oxalate and phosphate complex Ca^{2+}, minimum estimates of the free Ca^{2+} concentration within intracellular Ca^{2+} stores can be obtained from the association constants of the two anions. Such estimates of $[Ca^{2+}]_s$ in sarcoplasmic reticulum suggested values around 0.3 mM[25] or 0.5 mM.[27] These arguments might also apply in non-muscle cells. However, as described above for phosphate (Fig. 5.2A), Ca^{2+} buffering by these anions is not only a function of the intra-luminal Ca^{2+} concentration, but also depends on the concentration of the anion itself. Thus, these extrapolations should be viewed with caution.

LOADING OF CA²⁺ STORES WITH CA²⁺-SENSITIVE FLUORESCENT DYES

Acetoxylmethyl esters of Ca^{2+} sensitive fluorescent dyes are now widely used to study the free $[Ca^{2+}]$ within the cytosol ($[Ca^{2+}]_c$). However, depending on cell type and loading conditions, a non-trivial amount of these dyes may partition to intracellular Ca^{2+}

stores. Recently, investigators have used this property to gain information on the free Ca^{2+} concentration within intracellular stores($[Ca^{2+}]_s$). In these experiments cells are loaded with acetoxylmethyl esters of a fluorescent dye and the cytosolic dye is then removed by permeabilization of the cell membrane (e.g. with digitonin). In studies using the high affinity Ca^{2+} indicator fura-2 (K_d for Ca^{2+} ~0.25 µM) it was found that the probe was saturated within filled Ca^{2+} stores.[31,32] As saturation of fura-2 occurs in the low micromolar range, this suggests an intra-luminal free Ca^{2+} concentration above 5 µM. One study, using the intermediate affinity Ca^{2+} indicator mag-fura-2 (K_d for Ca^{2+} ~50 µM), measured astonishingly low $[Ca^{2+}]_s$ values of approximately 100 µM.[33] However, since the fluorescence of these probes is affected by protein binding, and mag-fura is also sensitive to Mg^{2+}, these values should be viewed with caution.

TARGETING OF AEQUORIN TO CA^{2+} STORES

A possibly promising approach to the measurement of $[Ca^{2+}]_s$ is the use of the Ca^{2+}-sensitive chemiluminescent protein aequorin. Cells, theoretically, can be transfected with the cDNA for aequorin, and, provided a proper targeting sequence can be defined, the protein could be directed specifically towards intracellular Ca^{2+} stores. Under these conditions, the chemiluminescence of the protein might give a good measure of $[Ca^{2+}]_s$ within the Ca^{2+} stores (for more details of this concept see ref. 6).

ARE THE NUMBER AND AFFINITY OF CALRETICULIN'S CA^{2+} BINDING SITES COMPATIBLE WITH A ROLE IN CA^{2+} STORAGE?

The calreticulin content of non-muscle tissues is between 50 and 500 µg/g of tissue or 1 and 10 µg/mg protein.[34] Thus, calreticulin is an extremely abundant protein, its contribution to the total cellular protein content possibly exceeding 0.1%. Consider liver, which has an approximate specific weight of 1.4 g/ml and a calreticulin content of 230 µg/g tissue.[34] From these data one may calculate that there are 320 mg calreticulin/liter of cell water, and since the molecular weight of calreticulin is 46-kDa, this corresponds to approximately 7 µmol calreticulin/liter of cell water. As each molecule of calreticulin has 20 low affinity Ca^{2+} binding sites and 1 high affinity Ca^{2+} binding site, the total Ca^{2+}

binding capacity of the calreticulin in liver should be around
0.15 mmol Ca²⁺/l cell water. Note that this estimate is somewhat
lower than a previous estimate, based on morphometric data, which
suggested a total Ca²⁺ binding capacity for liver calreticulin of approximately 0.5-1 mmol/l.[14]

How do these numbers relate to Ca²⁺ storage within the cell?
The amount of Ca²⁺ that will be bound to calreticulin in vivo is,
of course, not simply determined by the total number of Ca²⁺ binding sites, but also by their affinity. Calreticulin has only one high
affinity binding site (K_d 1-2 μM), alongside approximately 20 relatively low affinity sites (K_d ~1 mM; for review see ref. 35). The
number of Ca²⁺ storage sites provided by calreticulin will, therefore, be a function of the free Ca²⁺ concentration within the intracellular stores. Figure 5.3 shows the amount of Ca²⁺ bound to
calreticulin as a function of [Ca²⁺]$_s$ for three different estimates of

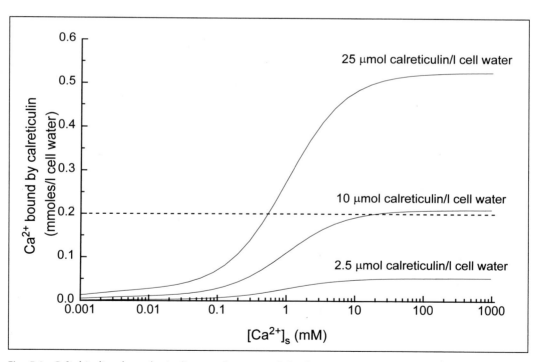

Fig. 5.3. Ca²⁺ binding by calreticulin as a function of the free Ca²⁺ concentration and the calreticulin
concentration within intracellular Ca²⁺ stores. The amount of Ca²⁺ bound to calreticulin in a cell (given as
mole/ liter of cell water) is shown as a function of the free Ca²⁺ concentration within intracellular Ca²⁺ stores.
The dashed line indicates the total amount of Ca²⁺ within intracellular stores (0.2 mmole/liter of cell water)
that was experimentally determined in PC12 cells.[21] Calreticulin was assumed to have 20 Ca²⁺ binding sites
with a K_d of 1 mM, and 1 Ca²⁺ binding site with a K_d of 1 μM.

cellular calreticulin content. These lines suggest that if $[Ca^{2+}]_s$ were in the millimolar range, Ca^{2+} binding to calreticulin might account for the bulk part of the intracellularly stored Ca^{2+} ($[Ca^{2+}]_{st}$ is approximately 0.2 mmole Ca^{2+}/l of cell water, see above). If, however, $[Ca^{2+}]_s$ were around 100 µM (as suggested by ref. 33), Ca^{2+} binding to calreticulin would account for only a relatively small fraction of the stored Ca^{2+}. Thus, clearly, the question "Is calreticulin a major contributor to Ca^{2+} storage within intracellular Ca^{2+} stores?" cannot be separated from the question "What is the free Ca^{2+} concentration within intracellular Ca^{2+} stores?"

DOES CALRETICULIN LOCALIZE TO CA²⁺ STORES?

Calreticulin appears to have a variety of functions at different cellular sites (see other chapters of this book) and would, therefore, not be expected to localize exclusively to intracellular Ca^{2+} stores. Previously, calreticulin has been suggested to act within the endoplasmic reticulum not only as a Ca^{2+} binding protein, but also as a molecular chaperone (see for example ref. 36), and, therefore, it might not localize exclusively to Ca^{2+} storage regions of the endoplasmic reticulum. In addition, other evidence indicates that calreticulin might be present in the cytosol,[37] in the nucleus,[38] and—at least in some cell types—within granules.[39] Despite these observations, an understanding of the spatial relationship between calreticulin, Ca^{2+} release sites (i.e. $Ins(1,4,5)P_3$ receptors and/or ryanodine receptors), and/or Ca^{2+} uptake sites (i.e. SERCA-type Ca^{2+}-ATPases) is crucial for our understanding of the potential role of calreticulin in cellular Ca^{2+} storage. For example, in muscle sarcoplasmic reticulum calsequestrin co-localizes with the ryanodine receptor (i.e. the terminal cysternae), but not with the Ca^{2+}-ATP-ase (i.e. the longitudinal sarcoplasmic reticulum). This suggests a deliberate increase in the Ca^{2+} storage capacity of the sarcoplasmic reticulum at Ca^{2+} release sites, via the specific localization of calsequestrin.[7]

The question of whether or not calreticulin co-localizes with other proteins involved in Ca^{2+} storage can be investigated in subcellular fractionation studies, in immunofluorescence studies, and in electron microscopy studies.

SUBCELLULAR FRACTIONATION STUDIES

Evidence for a co-localization of calreticulin with the $Ins(1,4,5)P_3$-sensitive Ca^{2+} release channel has been obtained in subcellular fractionation studies, using HL-60 promyelocytes[40] and rat liver.[41] Both studies reported a good correlation between the specific content of calreticulin and the $Ins(1,4,5)P_3$ receptor in various subcellular fractions, and also—at least partially—a separation of calreticulin from more general endoplasmic reticulum markers such as sulfatase C, NADPH cytochrome C reductase, and glucose-6-phosphatase. A discrepancy between the distribution of calreticulin and general endoplasmic reticulum markers would be compatible with specialized Ca^{2+} handling regions within the endoplasmic reticulum. In addition, in subcellular fractions from rabbit optic nerve and from rat brain, the distribution of calreticulin and SERCA2 were found to differ.[42] In contrast, in subcellular fractions of rat cerebellum, calreticulin co-sedimented with Ca^{2+}-ATPase activity, and with general endoplasmic reticulum markers (e.g. BiP), but with neither the $Ins(1,4,5)P_3$ receptor nor the ryanodine receptor.[43]

IMMUNOFLUORESCENCE STUDIES

In the muscle precursor cell line L6, a partial co-localization of calreticulin and Ca^{2+}-ATPase (SERCA2) was observed. The subcellular distribution of calreticulin immunofluorescence seemed to be larger than the area that was recognized by rough endoplasmic reticulum antibodies and extended towards the periphery of the cell. The Ca^{2+}-ATPase immunofluorescence partially overlapped that of calreticulin, but localized, in addition, to distinct vesicular structures.[44] In eggs of sea urchins and *Xenopus laevis*, both the $Ins(1,4,5)P_3$ receptor and calreticulin appeared to be evenly distributed throughout the endoplasmic reticulum.[45]

Immunofluorescence studies during phagocytosis in human neutrophils revealed a more dynamic picture:[46] calreticulin and SERCA2 were evenly distributed in non-phagocytosing neutrophils, but accumulated in the periphagosomal space during phagocytosis. Unpublished observations from our group suggest a similar behavior of the type I $Ins(1,4,5)P_3$ receptor. This apparent parallel redistribution of calreticulin with two proteins that are functionally involved in intracellular Ca^{2+} storage supports the suggestion that all three proteins are co-localized. However, in contrast, immunofluorescence studies in rhesus monkey brain suggested a differential distribution of calreticulin and Ca^{2+}-ATPase (SERCA2).[42]

ELECTRON MICROSCOPY STUDIES

Very few studies have addressed the question of whether or not calreticulin co-localizes with other proteins involved in Ca^{2+} homeostasis on an ultrastructural level. In one of these, in smooth muscle fibers, calreticulin appeared to be evenly distributed throughout the rough and the smooth endoplasmic reticulum, while calsequestrin and the Ins(1,4,5)P$_3$ receptor were preferentially found within peripheral smooth surfaced elements.[47]

In summary, the data presently available do not allow any clear-cut conclusion about the localization of calreticulin with respect to intracellular Ca^{2+} uptake and/or Ca^{2+} release sites. While some results suggest that calreticulin is evenly distributed throughout the endoplasmic reticulum, others suggest that it is concentrated at Ca^{2+} handling sites. Further, while some results suggest co-localization with Ins(1,4,5)P$_3$ receptors and/or Ca^{2+}-ATPases, others find a differential distribution. Tissue-specific differences are possible, but have not yet been proven. Clearly, as calreticulin is an intra-luminal endoplasmic reticulum protein without transmembrane segments, its concentration at Ca^{2+} handling sites would necessitate binding to membrane elements. Interestingly, calreticulin-binding proteins within the endoplasmic reticulum membrane have been described.[48] In addition, alongside retrieval through its C-terminal KDEL sequence, calreticulin appears to be retained within the endoplasmic reticulum through other, hitherto unknown, mechanisms.[49] Thus, it is possible that only a portion of calreticulin is freely diffusible within the endoplasmic reticulum, while another portion is membrane bound (and possibly kept in the proximity of Ca^{2+}-handling proteins). If this were the case, the distribution of calreticulin would then depend on the relative amounts of membrane-bound versus freely diffusible calreticulin.

DOES MODIFICATION OF CELLULAR CALRETICULIN CONTENT CHANGE CELLULAR CA^{2+} STORAGE?

Very few studies have reported the successful modification of cellular calreticulin content by knock-out or overexpression. This may reflect technical difficulties related to the fact that calreticulin, in addition to its presumed involvement in intracellular Ca^{2+} signaling, appears to be involved in other essential cellular processes (see other chapters in this book). However, two studies have found a correlation between cellular calreticulin content and cellular Ca^{2+}

storage. In studies using calreticulin anti-sense nucleotides it was reported that a decrease in cellular calreticulin content was paralleled by a decrease in the size of agonist-sensitive Ca^{2+} stores, as well as by an increased sensitivity of cells to Ca^{2+}-mediated cytotoxicity.[50] In other studies, it was found that the activation of T-lymphocytes leads to an approximately 2.5-fold increase in cellular calreticulin content, as well as to a 3-fold increase in intracellularly stored Ca^{2+}. However, the increased Ca^{2+} storage occurred predominantly in agonist-insensitive Ca^{2+} stores.[51]

CONCLUSION

This review of the seemingly simple question "Is calreticulin involved in cellular Ca^{2+} storage?" clearly highlights one of the weakest points in our knowledge of intracellular Ca^{2+} homeostasis. While cytosolic free Ca^{2+} concentration is being intensely investigated and increasingly understood (thanks to Ca^{2+}-sensitive fluorescent dyes, patch-clamp techniques and other technical developments), the stored Ca^{2+} concentration, and its regulation, remain a blind spot. We badly need reliable techniques to measure the free Ca^{2+} concentration within intracellular stores, as well as new approaches to investigate the geometry of these stores. Currently, the available data are compatible with a role for calreticulin in intracellular Ca^{2+} storage, but do not prove it. Table 5.1 illustrates two alternative scenarios: depending on the $[Ca^{2+}]_s$, calreticulin might make only a small contribution to total Ca^{2+} storage by a cell, or it might be a major player.

Recently, it has become increasingly clear that the $[Ca^{2+}]_s$ within intracellular stores is not only relevant for the regulation of cytosolic free Ca^{2+} concentration, but that it may also be a cellular signal in its own right. $[Ca^{2+}]_s$ has been implicated in the regulation of Ca^{2+} influx across the plasma membrane,[52] in the regulation of protein[53] and phospholipid[54] synthesis, and in the regulation of cellular growth.[54] To explain this signaling through $[Ca^{2+}]_s$, Ca^{2+}-binding proteins in the lumen of the endoplasmic reticulum would be necessary as sensors of $[Ca^{2+}]_s$, comparable, for example, with the role of calmodulin as a sensor of $[Ca^{2+}]_c$. Thus, the relationship between calreticulin and $[Ca^{2+}]_s$ might go beyond the "buffering" discussed in this chapter: calreticulin might also be a downstream mediator of $[Ca^{2+}]_s$ signals.

Table 5.1 Impact of the free Ca^{2+} concentration within intracellular stores on the possible relevance of calreticulin as a Ca^{2+} storage protein

	scenario 1	scenario 2
free $[Ca^{2+}]$ within stores $([Ca^{2+}]_s)$	5 mM	100 μM
total $[Ca^{2+}]$ within stores $([Ca^{2+}]_{st})$	25 mM	25 mM
store calreticulin concentration	1 mM	1 mM
calreticulin Ca^{2+}-binding sites within stores	21 mM	21 mM
bound $[Ca^{2+}]$ within stores	20 mM	24.9 mM
$[Ca^{2+}]$ bound to calreticulin	17.7 mM	2.8 mM
$[Ca^{2+}]$ bound to other store buffers	2.3 mM	22.1 mM
calreticulin saturation	84.3%	13.3%
calreticulin contribution to Ca^{2+} storage	70.8%	11.2%

Calculations were performed assuming a cell with a calreticulin concentration of 1 mM within the lumen of intracellular stores, and a total store Ca^{2+} concentration of 25 mM. These are estimates within the range suggested by the presently available data (see text). The calculations of calreticulin Ca^{2+}-binding sites are based on 20 low affinity sites of calreticulin (K_d=1 mM), and 1 high affinity site (K_d=1 μM). [35] The free $[Ca^{2+}]$ within the stores will then determine i) the total amount of Ca^{2+} bound within intracellular Ca^{2+} stores; ii) the amount of Ca^{2+} bound to calreticulin; iii) the amount of Ca^{2+} bound to other buffers within intracellular Ca^{2+} stores; iv) the % saturation of calreticulin (100 x Ca^{2+} bound to calreticulin/total number of calreticulin binding sites) and v) the % contribution of calreticulin to total cellular Ca^{2+} storage (100 x $[Ca^{2+}]$ bound to calreticulin/ total $[Ca^{2+}]$ within stores).

ACKNOWLEDGMENTS

This research was supported by grants from the Swiss National Foundation (32 30161.90), from the Carlos-and-Elsie-de-Reuter-Foundation, Geneva, from the Sandoz foundation, Basel, the Ernst-and-Lucie-Schmidheiny-Foundation, Geneva and from the Société Académique, Geneva.

REFERENCES

1. Somlyo AP. Cellular site of calcium regulation. Nature 1984; 308:516-517.
2. Carafoli E. Intracellular calcium homeostasis. Ann Rev Biochem 1987; 56:395-433.
3. Koch GLE. The endoplasmic reticulum and Ca^{2+} storage. BioEssays 1990; 12:527-531.
4. Rossier MF, Putney JWJ. The identity of the calcium storing, inositol 1,4,5-trisphosphate-sensitive organelle in non muscle cells: calciosome, endoplasmic reticulum, or both? TINS 1991; 14:310-314.
5. Krause KH. Ca^{2+} storage organelles. FEBS Lett 1991; 285:225-229.
6. Pozzan T, Rizzuto R, Volpe P et al. Molecular and cellular physiology of intracellular calcium stores. Physiol Rev 1994; 74:595-636.
7. MacLennan DH, Campbell KP, Reithmeier RAF. Calsequestrin. In: Cheng E. ed. Calcium and cell function. Academic Press. Inc 1983; 151-173.
8. Fliegel L, Ohnishi M, Carpenter MR et al. Amino acid sequence of rabbit fast-twitch skeletal muscle calsequestrin deduced from cDNA and peptide sequencing. Proc Natl Acad Sci USA 1987; 84:1167-1171.
9. Volpe P, Alderson-Lang BH, Madeddu L et al. Calsequestrin, a component of the inositol 1,3,5-trisphosphate-sensitive Ca^{2+} store of chicken cerebellum. Neuron 1990; 5:713-721.
10. Milner RE, Famulski KS, Michalak M. Calcium binding proteins in the sarcoplasmic/endoplasmic reticulum of muscle and nonmuscle cells. Mol Cell Biochem 1992; 112:1-13.
11. Macer DRJ, Koch GLE. Identification of a set of calcium-binding proteins in reticuloplasm, the luminal content of the endoplasmic reticulum. J Cell Sci 1988; 91:61-70.
12. Volpe P, Krause KH, Hashimoto S et al. Calciosome, a cytoplasmic organelle: the inositol 1,4,5-trisphosphate-sensitive Ca^{2+} store of nonmuscle cells. Proc Natl Acad Sci USA 1988; 85:1091-1095.
13. Krause KH, Simmerman KB, Jones LR et al. Sequence similarity of calreticulin with a Ca^{2+}-binding protein that copurifies with an Ins(1,4,5)P₃-sensitive Ca^{2+} store in HL-60 cells. Biochem J 1990; 270:545-548.
14. Treves S, De Mattei M, Lanfredi M et al. Calreticulin is a candidate for a calsequestrin-like function in Ca^{2+}-storage compartments (calciosomes) of liver and brain. Biochem J 1990; 271:473-480.
15. Van PN, Peter F, Söling H-D. Four intracisternal calcium-binding glycoproteins from rat liver microsomes with high affinity for calcium. J Biol Chem 1989; 264:17494-17501.
16. Fliegel L, Burns K, MacLennan DH et al. Molecular cloning of the high affinity calcium-binding protein (calreticulin) of skeletal muscle sarcoplasmic reticulum. J Biol Chem 1989; 264:21522-21528.

17. Smith MJ, Koch GLE. Multiple zones in the sequence of calreticulin (CRP55, calregulin, HACBP), a major calcium binding ER/SR protein. EMBO J 1989; 8:3581-3586.

18. Tharin S, Dziak E, Michalak M et al. Widespread tissue distribution of rabbit calreticulin, a non-muscle functional analogue of calsequestrin. Cell Tissue Res 1992; 269:29-37.

19. Baksh S, Michalak M. Expression of calreticulin in *Escherichia coli* and identification of its Ca^{2+} binding domains. J Biol Chem 1991; 286:21458-21465.

20. Neher E, Augustine GJ. Calcium gradients and buffers in bovine chromaffine cells. J Physiol (Lond) 1992; 450:273-301.

21. Fasolato C, Zottini M, Clementi E et al. Intracellular Ca^{2+} pools in PC12 cells. Three intracellular pools are distinguished by their turnover and mechanisms of Ca^{2+} accumulation, storage and release. J Biol Chem 1991; 266:20159-20167.

22. Meldolesi J, Madeddu L, Pozzan T. Intracellular Ca^{2+} storage organelles in non-muscle cells: heterogeneity and functional assignment. Biochim Biophys Acta 1990; 1055:130-140.

23. Somlyo AP, Bond M, Somlyo AV. Calcium content of mitochondria and endoplasmic reticulum in liver frozen rapidly in vivo. Nature 1985; 314:622-625.

24. Baumann O, Walz B, Somlyo AV et al. Electron probe microanalysis of calcium release and magnesium uptake by endoplasmic reticulum in bee photoreceptors. Proc Natl Acad Sci USA 1995; 88:741-744.

25. Inesi G, De Meis L. Regulation of steady state filling in sarcoplasmic reticulum: Roles of back-inhibition, leakage, and slippage of the calcium pump. J Biol Chem 1989; 264:5929-5936.

26. Fulceri R, Bellomo G, Gamberucci A, et al. Physiological concentrations of inorganic phosphate affect MgATP-dependent Ca^{2+} storage and inositol trisphosphate-induced Ca^{2+} efflux in microsomal vesicles from non-hepatic cells. Biochem J 1993; 289:299-906.

27. Martonosi A, Feretos R. Sarcoplasmic Reticulum 1. The uptake of Ca^{2+} by sarcoplasmic reticulum fragments. J Biol Chem 1964; 239:648-658.

28. Ghosh TK, Mullaney JM, Tarazi FI et al. GTP-activated communication between distinct inositol 1,4,5- trisphosphate-sensitive and -insensitive calcium pools. Nature 1989; 340:236-239.

29. Milner RE, Baksh S, Shemanko C et al. Calreticulin, and not calsequestrin, is the major calcium binding protein of smooth muscle sarcoplasmic reticulum and liver endoplasmic reticulum. J Biol Chem 1991; 266:7155-7165.

30. Pietrobon D, Di Virgilio F, Pozzan T. Structural and functional aspects of calcium homeostasis in eukaryotic cells. Eur J Biochem 1990; 193:599-622.

31. Short AD, Klein MG, Schneider MF et al. Inositol 1,4,5-trisphosphate-mediated quantal Ca²⁺ release measured by high resolution imaging of Ca²⁺ within organelles. J Biol Chem 1993; 268:25887-25893.

32. Glennon MC, St.J.Bird G, Kwan C-Y et al. Actions of vasopressin and the Ca²⁺-ATPase inhibitor, thapsigargin, on Ca²⁺ signaling in hepatocytes. J Biol Chem 1992; 267:8230-8233.

33. Hofer AM, Machen TE. Technique for in situ measurement of calcium in intracellular inositol 1,4,5-trisphosphate-sensitive stores using the fluorescent indicator mag-fura-2. Proc Natl Acad Sci USA 1993; 90:2598-2602.

34. Khanna NC, Waisman DM. Development of a radioimmunoassay for quantitation of calregulin in bovine tissues. Biochemistry 1986; 25:1078-1082.

35. Michalak M, Milner RE, Burns K et al. Calreticulin. Biochem J 1992; 285:681-692.

36. Nauseef WM, McCormick SJ, Clark RA. Calreticulin functions as a molecular chaperone in the biosynthesis of myeloperoxidase. J Biol Chem 1995; 270:4741-4747.

37. Dedhar S. Novel functions for calreticulin: Interaction with integrins and modulation of gene expression. TIBS 1994; 19:269-271.

38. Burns K, Atkinson EA, Bleackley RC et al. Calreticulin: From Ca²⁺ binding to control of gene expression. TICB 1994; 4:152-154.

39. Dupuis M, Schaerer E, Krause K-H et al. The calcium-binding protein calreticulin is a major constituent of lytic granules in cytolytic T lymphocytes. J Exp Med 1993; 177:1-7.

40. Van Delden C, Favre C, Spat A et al. Purification of an inositol 1,4,5-trisphosphate-binding calreticulin-containing intracellular compartment of HL-60 cells. Biochem J 1992; 281:651-656.

41. Enyedi P, Szabadkai G, Krause KH et al. Inositol 1,4,5-trisphosphate binding sites copurify with the putative Ca-storage protein calreticulin in rat liver. Cell Calcium 1993; 14:485-492.

42. Johnson RJ, Pyun HY, Lytton J et al. Differences in the subcellular localization of calreticulin and organellar Ca²⁺-ATPase in neurons. Mol Brain Res 1993; 17:9-16.

43. Nori A, Villa A, Podini P et al. Intracellular Ca²⁺ stores of rat cerebellum: heterogeneity within and distinction from endoplasmic reticulum. Biochem J 1993; 291:199-204.

44. Arber S, Krause KH, Caroni P. s-Cyclophilin is retained intracellularly via a unique COOH-terminal sequence and colocalizes with the calcium storage protein calreticulin. J Cell Biol 1992; 116:113-125.

45. Parys JB, McPherson SM, Mathews L et al. Presence of inositol 1,4,5-trisphosphate receptor, calreticulin, and calsequestrin in eggs of sea urchins and *Xenopus laevis*. Dev Biol 1994; 161:466-476.

46. Stendahl O, Krause KH, Krischer J et al. Redistribution of intracellular Ca^{2+} stores during phagocytosis in human neutrophils. Science 1994; 265:1439-1441.

47. Villa A, Podini P, Panzeri MC et al. The endoplasmic-sarcoplasmic reticulum of smooth muscle: Immunocytochemistry of vas deferens fibers reveals specialized subcompartments differently equipped for the control of Ca^{2+} homeostasis. J Cell Biol 1993; 121:1041-1051.

48. Burns K, Michalak M. Interactions of calreticulin with proteins of the endoplasmic and sarcoplasmic reticulum membranes. FEBS Lett 1993; 318:181-185.

49. Sönnichsen B, Füllekrug J, Van PN et al. Retention and retrieval: Both mechanisms cooperate to maintain calreticulin in the endoplasmic reticulum. J Cell Sci 1994; 107:2705-2717.

50. Liu N, Fine RE, Simons E et al. Decreasing calreticulin expression lowers the Ca^{2+} response to bradykinin and increases sensitivity to ionomycin in NG-108-15 cells. J Biol Chem 1994; 269:28635-28639.

51. Clementi E, Martino G, Grimaldi LME et al. Intracellular Ca^{2+} stores of T lymphocytes: changes induced by in vitro and in vivo activation. Eur J Immunol 1994; 24:1365-1371.

52. Putney JW Jr, Bird StJG. The signal for capacitative calcium entry. Cell 1993; 75:199-201.

53. Wong WL, Brostrom MA, Kuznetsov G et al. Inhibition of protein synthesis and early protein processing by thapsigargin in cultured cells. Biochem J 1993; 289:71-79.

54. Pelassy C, Breittmayer JP, Aussel C. Agonist-induced inhibition of phosphatidylserine synthesis is secondary to the emptying of intracellular Ca^{2+} stores in Jurkat T-cells. Biochem J 1992; 288:785-789.

55. Short AD, Bian J, Ghosh TK et al. Intracellular Ca^{2+} pool content is linked to control of cell growth. Proc Natl Acad Sci USA 1993; 90:4986-4990.

CHAPTER 6

CALRETICULIN AND THE MODULATION OF GENE EXPRESSION

Nasrin Mesaeli

INTRODUCTION

In 1991 Rojiani et al[1] made an unexpected discovery while studying the function of integrins: they showed that calreticulin interacts, in vitro, with the cytoplasmic domain of the α-subunit of integrin. The cytoplasmic domain of all integrin α-subunits contains a conserved amino acid sequence KGLFFKR. Rojiani et al[1] postulated that this amino acid sequence may be involved in a common signaling pathway that occurs via the α-subunit of integrins.

The authors used KGLFFKR-peptide affinity chromatography to identify proteins that interact with this specific amino acid sequence. A 60-kDa protein (designated p60) bound to the KGLFFKR-affinity matrix in a Ca^{2+}-dependent manner, and analysis of its N-terminal amino acid sequence revealed that it was calreticulin.[1] The significance of this observation is not clear, since localization of calreticulin to the cytoplasm has not been confirmed (Chapter 3). However, calreticulin does have profound effects on the adhesion properties of cells.[2]

We decided to search sequences in the Genbank for the KxFFKR amino acid motif, in order to determine whether other proteins contain either the KGLFFKR sequence or variations of it. To our surprise the first series of amino acid sequences matching this motif belonged to the family of steroid hormone receptors. This observation contributed to the hypothesis that calreticulin could perhaps interact with these receptors, thereby modulating steroid-sensitive gene expression. The KxFFKR amino acid sequence is found in the DNA binding domain (DBD) of all members of the nuclear hormone receptor superfamily (Table 6.1). At about the same time, in collaboration with Dr. M. Opas, we observed nuclear staining with anti-calreticulin antibodies suggesting that calreticulin might appear in the nucleus.[3]

Early in 1992, in collaboration with members of Chris Bleackley's laboratory, we set out to determine whether calreticulin could interact with the DBD of glucocorticoid receptors and modulate their function. A year later we learned that Dedhar et al had begun to investigate similar interactions between calreticulin and the DBD of the androgen receptor. In this chapter I have reviewed these studies, along with possible explanations for their observations, in detail.

STEROID HORMONE RECEPTORS

Members of the family of nuclear receptors are functionally and structurally related and include receptors for; steroid hormones (such as progesterone, androgen, estrogen and glucocorticoids); vitamins A and D; thyroid hormone and retinoic acid; and a group of receptors without known ligands, the "orphan" receptors.[4-8] These receptors play crucial roles in development, differentiation and homeostasis by mediating responses to extra- and intra-cellular stimuli. Functionally, they are ligand-dependent transcription factors that control diverse cellular processes by regulating the expression of their target genes. This regulation occurs via an interaction with specific DNA response elements associated with the genes.[4-8] The receptors themselves (transcription factors) are subject to post-transcriptional regulatory strategies that modulate their subcellular distribution, abundance, DNA-binding capacity, and function. For example, steroid receptors in the cytoplasm are found in multi-component complexes with other proteins, including the heat shock proteins hsp90, hsp70 and hsp56.[4-8] Ligand-binding facilitates dissociation of the receptors from these complexes, with subsequent nuclear translocation and binding to response sites.[4-8]

Table 6.1. Calreticulin binding amino acid sequence in the DBD of the nuclear receptor superfamily

Amino acid sequence	Origin	Receptor
K-V-F-F-K-R	Human	Glucocorticoid receptor
K-G-F-F-R-R	Human	Thyroid hormone receptor β
K-G-F-F-R-R	Human	Retinoic acid receptor α
K-G-F-F-R-R	Human	Retinoic acid receptor β
K-A-F-F-K-R	Human	Oestrogen receptor
K-V-F-F-K-R	Human	Progesterone receptor
K-V-F-F-K-R	Human	Mineralocorticoid receptor
K-V-F-F-K-R	Human	Androgen receptor
K-G-F-F-R-R	Human	Vitamin D receptor
K-G-F-F-K-R	Human	Retinoic acid receptor γ
K-G-F-F-K-R	Mouse	Thyroid hormone receptor α
K-G-F-F-R-R	Chicken	Thyroid hormone receptor β
K-G-F-F-R-R	Chicken	Thyroid hormone receptor α
K-G-F-F-R-R	Xenopus	Thyroid hormone receptor α
K-G-F-F-R-R	Xenopus	Thyroid hormone receptor α
K-G-F-F-R-R	Xenopus	Thyroid hormone receptor β
K-G-F-F-R-R	Xenopus	Thyroid hormone receptor β
K-G-F-F-R-R	Xenopus	Retinoic acid receptor α
K-G-F-F-R-R	Xenopus	Retinoic acid receptor γ
K-G-F-F-R-R	*Drosophila*	Ecdysone receptor

The consensus amino acid sequence K-x-F-F-(K/R)-R is found between the two zinc fingures in the DBD of all steroid hormone receptors. The amino acid sequences are taken from ref. 5.

Steroid receptors can be divided into three structural domains: the N-terminal domain, the DNA binding domain (DBD) in the central, basic region of the molecule, and the ligand binding domain at the C-terminus.[6] The N-terminal domain is the least conserved, and can vary in length from approximately 600 amino acids for the mineralocorticoid receptor to approximately 25 amino acids for the vitamin D receptor.[6] Importantly, each domain retains its function when fused to other proteins.[4] For example, fusion proteins expressed in *E. coli* that contain the glucocorticoid receptor DBD exhibit sequence-specific binding to the glucocorticoid response element (GRE).[9,10]

The DBD of nuclear receptors is organized into two zinc finger motifs, as schematically illustrated in Figure 6.1.[9,11] This region is highly conserved and contains sequences that are invariant among all members of the family, including the sequence KxFF($^K/_R$)R which is situated between the two zinc fingers. X-ray crystallography analysis of the glucocorticoid receptor DBD complexed with the GRE revealed that the peptide KVFFKR is in an α-helix conformation and is in direct contact with DNA.[11] It has been proposed that other members of the nuclear receptor family interact with their hormone response elements in a similar manner, via association of the DNA with their KxFFKR peptides.[12]

CALRETICULIN BINDS TO THE DNA BINDING DOMAIN OF STEROID HORMONE RECEPTORS

IN VITRO STUDIES

An interaction between calreticulin and the DBD of steroid receptors was first demonstrated, in vitro, by affinity chromatography[13] and co-immunoprecipitation.[14] Furthermore, DNA gel mobility shift assays revealed that this interaction prevents both the glucocorticoid receptor[13] and the androgen receptor[14] from interacting with their DNA response elements. Similar findings were recently confirmed for the vitamin D receptor[15] and the peroxisome proliferator-activated receptor (PPAR),[16] again using DNA gel mobility shift assays. Inclusion of the synthetic peptide KVFFKR in the assay reduces calreticulin's ability to inhibit interaction between the receptor and the DNA, suggesting that calreticulin interacts with this amino acid sequence in the DBD of these steroid hormone receptors (Fig. 6.1).

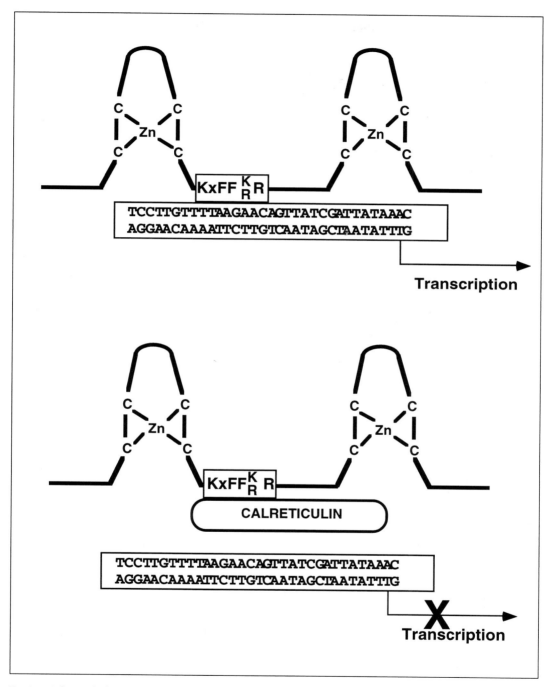

Fig. 6.1. Calreticulin binds to the DBD of steroid hormone receptors and prevents their interaction with DNA. The two zinc fingers of the DBD of a steroid receptor are shown. Calreticulin binds to the consensus amino acid sequence KxFF(K/R)R (see Table 6.1). Reprinted with permission from Burns K, Atkinson EA, Bleackley RC et al. TICB 1994; 4:152-154.

IN VIVO STUDIES

In order to determine whether similar interactions could occur in vivo, transient transfection experiments were carried out using a reporter gene under the control of promoters containing either the GRE[13] or the ARE.[14] As expected, steroid-sensitive expression of the reporter gene was inhibited in cells also transfected with calreticulin expression vectors.[13,14] Furthermore, overexpression of calreticulin in L fibroblasts inhibits dexamethasone-sensitive expression of the cytochrome p450 gene.[13] In a P19 embryonic carcinoma cell line that was selected for calreticulin over-expression, retinoic acid-sensitive expression of specific differentiation-markers was also suppressed.[14] In other studies the over-expression of calreticulin, in McAH-7777 hepatocytes, was found to inhibit dexamethasone-sensitive expression of the tyrosine aminotranferase gene but to have no effect on cAMP-dependent activation of the gene (Burns K, Opas M, Michalak M, submitted for publication). Further, in a rat osteoblast cell line (ROS 17/2.8) overexpression of calreticulin inhibited the transcriptional activation of a vitamin D-sensitive reporter gene by 1,25-dihydroxyvitamin D_3.[15]

Currently, evidence suggests that not all nuclear and steroid hormone receptors might be affected by overexpression of calreticulin. Winrow et al[16] found that, under the transient transfection conditions, over-expression of calreticulin in BSC40 cells had little or no effect on PPAR/RXR-mediated activation of a luciferase reporter gene controlled by the AOx-PPRE. Nevertheless, as mentioned above, calreticulin interacts with the PPAR in vitro and inhibits its binding to DNA. Additional studies are required, both in vivo and in vitro, to clarify the specificity of these interactions.

HOW DOES CALRETICULIN INHIBIT TRANSCRIPTIONAL ACTIVATION BY STEROID HORMONE RECEPTORS IN VIVO?

As illustrated in Figure 6.1, in vitro the binding of calreticulin to the KxFFKR amino acid sequence of the steroid receptor would mask the DBD, thus preventing its interaction with the binding element of the DNA. It is not clear whether the same mechanism is responsible for calreticulin's in vivo effects on steroid-sensitive gene expression. If calreticulin does interact with the DBD of steroid hormone receptors in vivo, these interactions could prevent the receptors from binding to their responsive elements on the DNA and/or affect their movement to the nucleus. However, in vivo, calreticulin may not interact directly with the DBD of steroid receptors at all, but may have other, indirect effects.

CAN CALRETICULIN INTERACT DIRECTLY WITH STEROID RECEPTORS IN VIVO?

Most steroid receptors are localized in the cytoplasm or nucleus of the cell, while calreticulin is resident in the endoplasmic reticulum. For calreticulin to interact directly with the DBD of steroid receptors in vivo, it would have to gain access to the cytoplasm and/or the nucleus.[17] This requirement is not readily reconciled with the observations that calreticulin is synthesized (i) with a signal sequence at its amino terminus and (ii) with the KDEL retention signal at its carboxyl terminus. These signals should result in an almost exclusive localization of calreticulin to the lumen of the endoplasmic reticulum.[17-19] Calreticulin does possesses a putative nuclear localization signal (NLS),[18] but, presumably, in order for this signal to target calreticulin to the nucleus, the protein would first have to gain access to the cytoplasm. Currently, despite major efforts in a number of laboratories, there is no convincing evidence for localization of calreticulin to the cytoplasm.

While most evidence indicates that calreticulin is localized to the lumen of the endoplasmic reticulum, there are a number of proteins known to localize to more than one intracellular compartment.[20] Danpure has presented a comprehensive review of the possible mechanisms by which the same protein might be targeted to different intracellular compartments.[20] There are a number of mechanisms by which calreticulin (or any other endoplasmic reticulum protein) could appear in the cytoplasm.[17] These include alternative transcription, leading to the synthesis of calreticulin without its N-terminal signal sequence, and alternative splicing of calreticulin mRNA. Post-translational modification and differential regulation of expression also play a role in the intracellular trafficking of proteins.[20] Presently there is no evidence that mRNA for calreticulin is alternatively spliced, or that alternative mechanisms for initiation of transcription and translation occur.[17] Calreticulin is encoded by a single, relatively simple and highly conserved gene.[21,22]

Under conditions of overexpression, calreticulin may well be inefficiently translocated into the endoplasmic reticulum, and therefore remain in the cytosol. This could occur either because the translocation apparatus is overloaded, or as a response to cellular stress. In support of the latter suggestion, there is an increase in the expression of calreticulin at the cell surface following infection of fibroblasts with cytomegalovirus.[23] There is currently no evidence that proteins move from the lumen of the endoplasmic reticulum to the cytoplasm. However, this possibility has been considered for certain bacterial toxins,[24] and although this appears to be an unlikely mechanism for the movement of calreticulin to the cytoplasm, there is presently no evidence to discount it. The suggestion that cleavage of the KDEL signal sequence could direct calreticulin to cytoplasm[25] is unlikely, as this form of the protein would be secreted from the cell. A novel possibility for the trafficking of calreticulin is that it could be targeted out of the endoplasmic reticulum in one cell and delivered, by exocytosis, into the cytoplasm of another cell. Calreticulin has been localized in the lytic granules of cytotoxic T lymphocytes,[26,27] and from here it could gain access to the cytoplasm of a target cell by direct injection. Obviously, further investigation with more sensitive tools (antibodies) and techniques is required to determine whether calreticulin is found, perhaps transiently and in small amounts, in the cytoplasm.

If calreticulin did appear in the cytoplasm, could it move to the nucleus? Hatcher's group has shown recently (Chapter 12) that calreticulin is transported to the nucleus of HUVEC cells under in vitro nuclear import conditions.[28] Further, we have detected transport of FITC-calreticulin to the nucleus of permeabilized fibroblasts (Burns K, Michalak M, unpublished observations), and FITC-labeled calreticulin, when micro-injected into fibroblasts, becomes transiently nuclear (Dzia E, Opas M, unpublished observations). Although these results indicate that cellular mechanisms allow the transport of "cytoplasmic calreticulin" to the nucleus, immunocytochemical and biochemical experiments indicate that calreticulin is not resident in the nucleus. Again, further investigation is required to determine whether or not any translocation of calreticulin to the nucleus occurs under physiological conditions.

DOES CALRETICULIN AFFECT STEROID-SENSITIVE GENE EXPRESSION INDIRECTLY?

Current evidence strongly suggests that, in vivo, calreticulin may not interact directly with the DBD of steroid receptors, but more likely inhibits their activation of transcription indirectly, from the lumen of the endoplasmic reticulum. The regulation of gene expression via "signals" from the endoplasmic reticulum has already been demonstrated, specifically for protein disulfide isomerase and BiP.[29,30] The transcription of genes encoding proteins resident in the endoplasmic reticulum is induced when unfolded proteins accumulate in the lumen. A transmembrane endoplasmic reticulum protein with serine/threonine kinase activity has been implicated in "sensing" these changes in the lumen, leading to the activation of a specific set of transcription factors.[29,30] Gene expression is apparently also regulated by ERp61, an endoplasmic reticulum protein that has recently been identified as a member of the family of protein disulfide isomerase proteins.[31] In leukemia cells from patients with chronic myelogenous leukemia, ERp61 has been demonstrated to alter complex formation between nuclear proteins and regulatory regions of interferon-inducible genes.[29]

Similar mechanism(s) may be involved in calreticulin-dependent inhibition of steroid-sensitive gene expression. When calreticulin is overexpressed it may bind to a transmembrane endoplasmic reticulum "receptor" causing "signal" transduction across the endoplasmic reticulum membrane. Alternatively, overexpression of calreticulin might alter the concentrations of Ca^{2+} in both the endoplasmic reticulum and cytoplasm. Fluctuations in the cytoplasmic concentration of Ca^{2+} may directly affect steroid hormone function. In addition, Greber and Gerace[32] have shown that depletion of Ca^{2+} from the lumen of the endoplasmic reticulum affects transport of molecules into the nucleus.

In conclusion, physiological conditions may exist in which calreticulin co-localizes with steroid hormone receptors in the cytoplasm, and/or in the nucleus, to modulate their function. More studies are required to investigate this possibility. Alternatively, the protein might affect steroid-sensitive gene expression indirectly, from within the lumen of the endoplasmic reticulum. Again further studies are required to determine whether this is the case. Certainly, investigation of the intracellular trafficking of calreticulin may help to explain how overexpression of this protein alters steroid hormone-sensitive gene transcription.

ACKNOWLEDGMENTS

The author is a recipient of a fellowship from the Heart and Stroke Foundation of Canada. I am grateful to R.E. Milner for critical reading of the manuscript.

REFERENCES

1. Rojiani MV, Finlay BB, Gray V et al. In vitro interaction of a polypeptide homologous to human Ro/SS-A antigen (calreticulin) with a highly conserved amino acid sequence in the cytoplasmic domain of integrin α subunits. Biochemistry 1991; 30:9859-9865.
2. Leung-Hagesteijn C, Milankov YK, Michalak M et al. Cell attachment to extracellular matrix substrates is inhibited upon downregulation of expression of calreticulin, an intracellular integrin α-subunit-binding protein. J Cell Sci 1994; 107:589-600.
3. Opas M, Dziak E, Fliegel L et al. Regulation of expression and intracellular distribution of calreticulin, a major calcium binding protein of non-muscle cells. J Cell Physiol 1991; 149:160-171.
4. Evans RM. The steroid and thyroid hormone receptor superfamily. Science 1988; 240:889-895.
5. Laudet V, Hänni C, Coll J et al. Evolution of the nuclear receptor gene superfamily. EMBO J 1991; 11:1003-1013.
6. Beato M. Gene regulation by steroid hormones. Cell 1989; 56:335-344.
7. Tsai M-J, O'Malley BW. Mechanism of steroid hormone regulation of gene transcription. Molecular Biology Intelligence Unit. R.G. Landes Company, Austin, USA. 1994.
8. Muller M, Renkawitz R. The glucocorticoid receptor. Biochim Biophys Acta 1991; 1088:171-182.
9. Freedman LP, Luisi BF, Korszun ZR et al. The function and structure of the metal coordination sites within the glucocorticoid receptor DNA-binding domain. Nature 1988; 334:543-546.
10. Evans RM, Hollenberg SM. Zinc fingers: gilt by association. Cell 1988; 52:1-3.
11. Luisi BF, Xu WX, Otwinowski Z et al. Crystallographic analysis of the interaction of the glucocorticoid receptor with DNA. Nature 1991; 352:497-505.
12. Schwabe JWR, Chapman L, Finch JT et al. The crystal structure of the estrogen receptor DNA-binding domain bound to DNA: How receptors discriminate between their response elements. Cell 1993; 75:567-578.
13. Burns K, Duggan B, Atkinson EA et al. Modulation of gene expression by calreticulin binding to the glucocorticoid receptor. Nature 1994; 367:476-480.

14. Dedhar S, Rennie PS, Shago M et al. Inhibition of nuclear hormone receptor activity by calreticulin. Nature 1994; 367:480-483.

15. Wheeler D, Horsford J, Michalak M et al. Calreticulin inhibits vitamin D3 signal transduction by blocking DNA binding of VDR/RXR heterodimers. Nucl Ac Res 1995; (submitted)

16. Winrow CJ, Miyata KS, Marcus SL et al. Calreticulin modulates the in vitro DNA binding but not the in vivo transcriptional activation by PPAR/RXR heterodimers. Mol Cell Endocrinol 1995; 111:175-179.

17. Burns K, Atkinson EA, Bleackley RC et al. Calreticulin: from Ca^{2+} binding to control of gene expression. TICB 1994; 4:152-154.

18. Michalak M, Milner RE, Burns K et al. Calreticulin. Biochem J 1992; 285:681-692.

19. Nash PD, Opas M, Michalak M. Calreticulin, not just another calcium-binding protein. Mol Cell Biochem 1994; 135:71-78.

20. Danpure CJ. How can the products of a single gene be localized to more than one intracellular compartment? TICB 1995; 5:230-238.

21. McCauliff DP, Yang YS, Wilson J et al. The 5' flanking sequence region of the human calreticulin gene shares homology with the human GRP78, GRP94 and protein disulfide isomerase promoters. J Biol Chem 1992; 267:2557-2562.

22. Waser M, Michalak M. Regulation of calreticulin gene expression by calcium. J Biol Chem 1995; (submitted)

23. Zhu JH, Newkirk MM. Viral induction of the human autoantigen calreticulin. Clin Invest Med 1994; 17:196-205.

24. Pelham RB, Roberts LM, Lord JM. Toxin entry: how reversible is the secretory pathway? TICB 1992; 2:183-185.

25. Dedhar S. Novel functions for calreticulin: interaction with integrins and modulation of gene expression? TIBS 1994; 19:269-271.

26. Dupuis M, Schaerer E, Krause KH et al. The calcium binding protein calreticulin is a major constituent of lytic granules in cytolytic T lymphocytes. J Exp Med 1993; 177:1-7.

27. Bleackley RC, Atkinson E, Burns K et al. Calreticulin: a granule protein by design by default? Curr Topics Microbiol Immunol 1995; 198:145-159.

28. Adam SA, Marr RS, Gerace L. Nuclear protein import in permeabilized mammalian cells requires soluble cytoplasmic factors. J Cell Biol 1990; 111:807-816.

29. Johnson E, Henzel W, Deisseroth A. An isoform of protein disulfide isomerase isolated from chronic myelogenous leukemia cells alters complex formation between nuclear proteins and regulatory regions of interferon-α inducible genes. J Biol Chem 1992; 267:14412-14417.

30. Cox JS, Shamu CE, Walter P. Transcriptional induction of genes encoding endoplasmic reticulum resident proteins requires a transmembrane protein kinase. Cell 1993: 73:1197-1206.

31. Lewis MJ, Mazzarella RA, Green M. Structure and assembly of the endoplasmic reticulum: Biosynthesis and intracellular sorting of ERp61, ERp59, and ERp49, three protein components of murine endoplasmic reticulum. Arch Biochem Biophys 1986; 245:389-403.
32. Greber UF, Gerace L. Depletion of calcium from the lumen of endoplasmic reticulum reversibly inhibits passive diffusion and signal-mediated transport into the nucleus. J Cell Biol 1995: 128:5-14.

CHAPTER 7

ROLE OF CALRETICULIN IN RUBELLA VIRUS REPLICATION

Chintamani D. Atreya, Gregory P. Pogue,
Nishi K. Singh and Hira L. Nakhasi

HOST-VIRUS INTERACTIONS

Viruses are intracellular pathogens which have evolved intricate relationships with their respective hosts. A successful virus infection includes the establishment of its replication cycle in an infected cell, dissemination to target tissue or cells, and occasional establishment of persistent infections. Each step in the infection process involves interplay between virally encoded nucleic acids and proteins and specific cellular proteins. In the case of viruses with DNA genomes, many important contributions by the host, from receptors to transcriptional factors, have been identified and have provided important insights into the normal functions of eukaryotic cells.[1] Recent investigations into RNA viruses have also identified important contributions from the host such as the nature of receptors for poliovirus,[2] measles virus[3] and Sindbis virus,[4] as well as insights into many events involving viral RNA synthesis and pathogenesis.[5,6] Further consequences of host-virus interactions includes requisite processing of viral antigens and stimulation of protective immune response against virions and infected cells. Recent contributions from various molecular virology laboratories undoubtedly suggest that host-virus interactions are pivotal in viral replication, pathogenesis and emerging disease aspects.[6-9]

Calreticulin, edited by Marek Michalak. © 1996 R.G. Landes Company.

Several cellular proteins have been identified that bind viral RNA sequences regulating RNA replication and translation. Often, these regulatory sequences contain stem loop (SL) structures. The RNA bacteriophage, Qβ, utilizes an RNA polymerase complex consisting of a phage encoded polymerase and three host-encoded proteins, a ribosomal protein and elongation factors Tu and Ts, which are normally involved in cellular mRNA translation.[10] Replication of several nonsegmented negative-strand RNA viruses such as vesicular stomatitis virus (VSV), mumps virus, parainfluenza virus (PIV) type 3 and Sendi virus also involves contributions from certain cellular factors.[11-14] In poliovirus, binding of ribosome-associated host cellular protein (p36) and a viral protein (3CD) to the clover leaf RNA structure present at the 5'- end of genomic RNA is thought to stimulate the initiation of virus RNA synthesis.[5] Aberrant poliovirus RNA translation in rabbit reticulocytes has been shown to be corrected by binding of the La antigen to a RNA stem-loop structure present in the viral 5' non-translational region.[15] La antigen was also shown to bind the human immunodeficiency virus type 1 (HIV-1) TAR element alleviating translational repression of HIV-1 mRNA by TAR sequences.[16,17] Recently, a sub-set of autoantigens have also been shown to bind the 5' leader sequence of rubella virus RNA and this binding is implicated in the stimulation of translation.[18] From these studies it is evident that a crucial interplay occurs between host factors and the replication and translation machinery of RNA viruses.

INTRODUCTION TO RUBELLA VIRUS

Our laboratory has been involved in defining the molecular events that occur during rubella virus (RV) replication and pathogenesis. RV, an enveloped virus, is the sole member of the rubivirus genus of the Togaviridae family, which also includes the alphaviruses.[19] RV is a major human pathogen and causative agent of German measles which appears as a mild rash and fever in children and young adults. However, RV infection during the first trimester of pregnancy can cause fetal death or multisystem birth defects, including deafness, cataracts, mental retardation, and congenital heart disease.[20] Histopathological analysis of the tissues of infants with congenital rubella syndrome revealed teratogenic effects, such as general retardation in growth due to mitotic inhibition.[21] In many natural and vaccine-derived infections, RV can establish and maintain persistent infections.[22] Approximately 15% of adult women contracting RV infections report joint related complications, such as arthropathy and arthritis.[22,23] From these cases, a significant number of individuals develop chronic arthritis causing long term discomfort.[23] An effective vaccine has been developed which has dramatically reduced the incidence of rubella infection.[23] In spite of its availability, a significant number of natural infections are reported each year and in addition, several cases of adverse reactions have been also reported following vaccination.[23] Further, in the last few years, the incidence of maternal infection and consequent congenital rubella syndrome has been on the rise.[24]

The causative agent of rubella infections consists of a virion containing a positive (+) sense 40S single-stranded polyadenylated genomic RNA (9,757 nucleotides in length) encapsidated within an lipid bilayer envelope presenting two virus encoded glycoproteins E1 and E2 (Fig. 7.1A).[25] The 5' proximal 6,615 nucleotides contain a long open reading frame (ORF) that encodes for two putative nonstructural proteins (Fig. 7.1B).[26] In the infected cells, a 24S subgenomic mRNA derived from the 3' end of genomic RNA is translated into a 110-kDa polypeptide precursor which is processed into capsid, E1 and E2 proteins (Fig. 7.1C).[27]

RUBELLA VIRUS REPLICATION

The general replication strategy of RV is similar to that of the alphaviruses (Fig. 7.1). Initiation of the virus replication cycle is mediated by entrance of the virion into the cell presumably by receptor-mediated endocytosis, although, to date, no receptor has been molecularly defined (Fig. 7.1A). Acidification of late endosomal compartments induces the fusion of the virion membrane with that of the endosome, thus allowing the release of the nucleocapsid containing the 40S genomic RNA into the cytoplasm (Fig. 7.1A). The non-structural proteins, including an RNA-dependent RNA-polymerase are translated from the 5' ORF of the genomic (+)-sense RNA (Fig. 7.1B). These proteins presumably associate with acesssory factors to form the viral replicase that initiates negative (-)-sense RNA synthesis from within the 3' poly-A tail (Fig. 7.1B-C). The (-) strand RNA intermediate is then used as a template for multiple rounds of either genomic or subgenomic RNA synthesis (Fig. 7.1C). The virion proteins are translated from the subgenomic RNA and, following post-translational

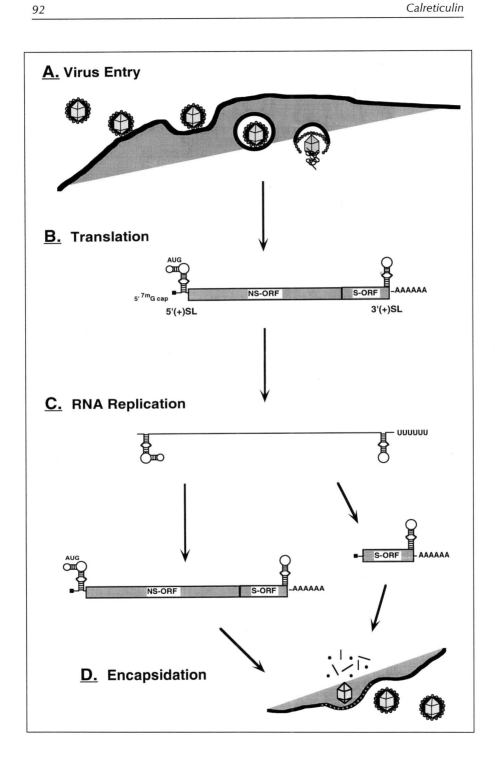

modifications in the endoplasmic reticulum and Golgi systems, the 40S RNA is encapsidated into a nucleocapsid (Fig. 7.1D). The virion then buds from the host cytoplasmic membrane, thus initiating a new cycle of virus replication.

Many lines of evidence have invoked the participation of host-encoded factors in several steps of RNA virus replication. The presence of numerous *cis*-acting elements of diverse sequence and structural contexts within a single virus genome suggests that the virus encoded RNA-dependent RNA-polymerases have little sequence specificity.[6] This, coupled with the relatively few non-structural proteins encoded by most RNA viruses, has led to the model that cellular proteins associate with virally-encoded polymerases and aid in the process of promoter sequence recognition and polymerase positioning.[6,7] This has been demonstrated in the case of the bacteriophage Qβ where translational elongation factors Tu and Ts, the components of the virus replicase, recognize the terminal sequences of the virus RNA allowing correct initiation in RNA synthesis.[10]

To explore possible host contributions to RV replication, accumulation of the viral products was analysed in cells incubated with several agents that inhibit different stages of cellular gene expression. One of the most instructive of these experiments involved treatment of Vero 76 cells, an African green monkey kidney derived cell line, with Actinomycin D.[28] Addition of Actinomycin D prior to, or during the initial hours of, RV infection (2 or 4 hours) reduced the synthesis of virion proteins or RV RNA by almost 10-fold when compared with control experiments without Actinomycin D (Fig. 7.2). In contrast, addition of

---

Fig. 7.1. (left) *Schematic representation of RV replication. A. Virion fuses with the cell membrane, enters cell by endocytic mechanisms and the virion dissembles releasing viral genomic RNA into cytoplasm. B. Using cellular translational machinery, viral RNA is translated to produce nonstructural proteins. C. Viral replicase, presumably composed of virus- and host-encoded proteins, associates with the 3' end of the genomic RNA to initiate antigenomic, negative (–), strand RNA synthesis. The resulting (–) strand RNA provides a template for the synthesis of multiple rounds of genomic (40S) and subgenomic (24S) RNAs by the replicase. The subgenomic RNA is translated into the viral structural proteins; some of which are presented on the cell surface following modification in the endoplasmic reticulum and Golgi apparatus. D. Viral genomic RNA and the structural proteins assemble at the cell membrane into mature virions which are then released into interstitial spaces. AUG, translation initiation codon for non-structural proteins; 5' and 3'(+) stem-loop (SL) RNA structures; NS-ORF, nonstructural protein coding sequence; S-ORF, structural protein coding region.*

Actinomycin D 8 hours following RV infection reduced the accumulation of most RV products by only ~60% (Fig. 7.2). Results from these experiments suggested that transcription of host-encoded RNAs was requisite for a successful RV infection. Further, these results significantly contrasted with the closely related alphaviruses where productive infections could be observed in cells treated with Actinomycin D prior to, or 2 or 4 hours post infection.[29] Thus, our studies suggested that RV replication has the peculiar requirement for host-encoded contributions.

IDENTIFICATION OF *CIS*-ACTING FUNCTION OF RV 5' AND 3'(+)SL STRUCTURES

As previously discussed, initiation of virus RNA synthesis involves the activity of a multi-component protein complex deemed the viral replicase. This complex includes both virus and host-encoded proteins that must interact with virus *cis*-acting sequences, presumably residing at the 5' or 3' terminal ends of the virus RNAs,

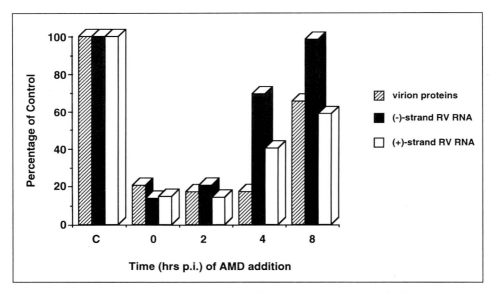

Fig. 7.2. Effect of Actinomycin D (AMD) mediated host transcriptional inhibition on RV replication. On X-axis, (C) indicates control cells receiving no Actinomycin D treatment, where accumulation levels of viral protein, (+) and (–) sense RNA production were assigned values of 100%. Levels of virus products, accumulated in RV infected cells treated at 0, 2, 4 or 8 hours post infection (hr p.i.) with Actinomycin D, were normalized with respect to controls and reported. Note, Actinomycin D had an inhibitory negative effect on RV infection as reflected in reduced accumulation of viral proteins and RNA. However, by 8 hr the level of (–) strand RNA products appeared virtually unaffected by Actinomycin D treatment.

and initiate RNA synthesis. Comparison of RNA sequences from wild-type as well as from several vaccine strains of rubella virus revealed a conserved sequence near the 3' end of virion RNA that can potentially form a stable SL structure under physiological conditions.[7,25] Comparison of the available 5' RV RNA sequences with that of closely related alphaviruses also suggested the presence of a conserved 5'(+)SL element.[18,25] Previously, from sequence analysis of a number of alphaviruses, Strauss and colleagues had hypothesized that conserved 5' and 3' sequence elements are important for alphavirus RNA replication.[30] Indeed, mutational analysis of sequences constituting the 5'(+)SL sequence and a 3' terminal 19 nucleotide motif of Sindbis virus indicated that these elements were critical for proper virus replication.[9] Further, the role of 5' and 3' sequence elements, as well as those promoting subgenomic RNA synthesis in Sindbis virus, were assessed using a defective interfering (DI) RNA as a replication template.[31] This approach allowed the performance of various mutant RNAs to be determined in infections containing the wild-type virus, that also provided a useful internal control. The use of a DI RNA allowed the construction and testing of lethal mutations, which in this context would not eliminate virus replication and thus allow the effects of all mutations to be quantitatively measured.

To elucidate the contributions of terminal SL sequences of RV RNA in replication, we took a similar approach to that described for Sindbis virus[31] and chose to construct artificial RV DI RNAs. Chimeric reporter constructs were designed to replace the normal RV coding regions with the chloramphenicol acetyltransferase (CAT) ORF (Fig. 7.1B).[7,18] The 5'(+)SL sequence from the RV genome was placed in frame with the CAT ORF and the 3' terminal 165 nts of the RV genome, which contains the 3'(+)SL structure and a poly-A tail, was then ligated to the 3' end of the CAT non-translated region.[7,18] Several mutations were then introduced into the RV SL regions to ascertain the contributions of these sequences to the translation and replication of RV genomic RNA. In summary, in vitro and in vivo studies revealed that both RV 5' and 3'(+)SL elements promote the translation of the CAT ORF; in particular, the 3'(+)SL appeared to have a secondary, enhancing function.[18] The 3'(+)SL sequence, however, was absolutely necessary for negative (-) strand RNA synthesis of the chimeric RV/CAT RNA in RV infected cells.[7] These results suggested that important *cis*-acting functions are performed by the 5' and 3'(+)SL sequences of RV RNA.

BINDING OF CELLULAR PHOSPHO PROTEINS TO THE RV 3'(+)SL RNA

The requirement of the 5' and 3'(+)SL RNA sequences for normal virus RNA functions suggested that they may be recognized by components of the virus replicase complex. Investigations into the replication of Qβ and poliovirus had suggested that host-encoded proteins may make essential contributions to the virus RNA replication.[5,10] The identification of additional examples of host-virus interactions therefore would contribute greatly to our knowledge of the molecular events necessary for RNA virus replication. For such reasons, we initiated studies to look for host protein interactions with the cis-acting elements of RV RNA. The RV 3'(+)SL (Fig. 7.1B and 7.1C) is absolutely required for (-) strand RNA synthesis to be initiated by the RV replicase.[7] To identify proteins specifically interacting with the 3'(+)SL, we synthesized radiolabeled RNA molecules encompassing the nucleotides of the this putative SL structure (Fig. 7.3C). These RNA probes were then incubated with cytosolic extracts isolated from mock- or RV-infected Vero 76 cells, and RNA-protein complexes formed were analyzed by RNA mobility shift and UV crosslinking procedures.[32] A single, specific RNA-protein complex was identified upon incubation of cytolysates from mock-infected cells with the 3'(+)SL RNA (Fig. 7.3A, lane 1). The intensity of this binding activity increased several fold in lysates derived from confluent cell cultures compared to extracts from actively dividing cells.[32] Incubation of lysates from RV-infected cells with the 3'(+)SL RNA resulted in a complex of similar mobility to that observed in uninfected cytolysates and additional specific RNA-protein complexes of slower mobility (Fig. 7.3A, lane 2). The larger RNA-protein complexes appeared 4-8 hours following RV infection, coinciding with the onset of detectable (-) strand RNA synthesis.[32] Treatment of RV infected cells with either transcription or translation inhibitors (AMD or cycloheximide) resulted in a significant delay in the emergence of the larger RNA-protein complexes.[32] Delay in formation of higher molecular weight RNA-protein complexes by addition of AMD corroborated our earlier studies showing AMD impairment of host protein expression dramatically

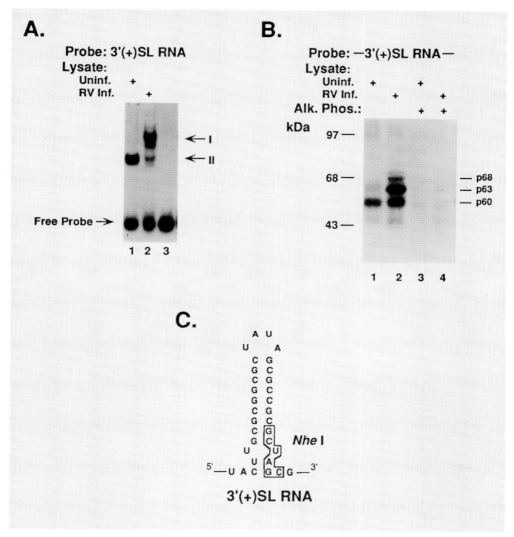

Fig. 7.3. Binding of cellular phosphoproteins to the RV 3'(+)SL RNA. A. Radiolabeled 3'(+)SL RNA was incubated with proteins present in cytolysates derived from uninfected (lane 1) and RV infected (lane 2) Vero 76 cells. Complexes were resolved in an RNA-mobility shift assay using non-denaturing conditions. Migration pattern of 3'(+)SL RNA in the absence of cellular proteins is shown in lane 3. The locations of slower migrating RNA-protein complexes are indicated by I and II. B. Analysis of proteins associated with RV 3'(+)SL RNA. Radiolabeled 3'(+)SL RNA was incubated with cytolysates derived from uninfected (lane 1) and RV infected (lane 2) Vero 76 cells, exposed to UV light to induce covalent linkages between closely associated RNA and protein components and products were then resolved by SDS-PAGE. Approximate molecular weights (kDa) for distinct labeled proteins are 60-, 63- and 68-kDa. Treatment of uninfected (lane 3) or RV infected cytolysates (lane 4) with alkaline phosphatase prior to incubation with radiolabeled 3'(+)SL RNA abrogated the formation of RNA protein complexes. C. The predicted structure of the RV 3'(+)SL RNA used as binding substrate is shown with the location of the unique Nhe I site present in its cDNA.

reduced RV replication (Fig. 7.2). Together, these data suggest that the induction of high affinity RNA binding activity by RV infection was not simply due to modifications of pre-existing proteins, but required new protein synthesis.

Treatment of uninfected cytolysates with UV light after mixing with radiolabeled 3'(+)SL RNA resulted in the transfer of label to a ~60-kDa protein (Fig. 7.3B, lane 1). Similar UV crosslinking studies using lysates from RV-infected cells revealed two additional proteins of ~63- and 68-kDa bound to the 3'(+)SL RNA (Fig. 7.3B, lane 2). The great increase in the binding activity seen following RV infections also could be due to post-translational modifications of proteins in addition to an increase in their synthesis. Phosphorylation of proteins has been shown to be an important step in the replication process of several virus systems,[33,34] and may determine whether a virus can replicate in a given cell type. Treatment of lysates with alkaline phosphatase resulted in abrogation of the binding of all proteins to the 3'(+)SL RNA (Fig. 7.3B, lanes 3-4), indicating that phospho-proteins were responsible for the binding activity. Since the 3' (+) SL RNA is the substrate for the RNA-protein complexes, we analyzed the RNA determinates required by the cellular proteins for binding. It was observed that a mutant 3'(+)SL RNA containing deletions of the two unpaired uridines in the RV 3' (+) SL RNA (Fig. 7.3C, bulge region) was unable to be bound by the cytosolic proteins.[32] Further, nucleotide substitutions for the unpaired uridines in the bulge domain of the 3'(+)SL RNA revealed that the cellular proteins bound the mutant probes with the following preference, UU>GG>AA>CC (Atreya, unpublished data). The profound effects of such subtle mutations demonstrate the high specificity with which the ~60-, 63- and 68-kDa cytosolic proteins bind the 3'(+)SL RNA.

IDENTIFICATION OF RV 3'(+)SL RNA BINDING PROTEIN AS CALRETICULIN

Since we demonstrated that host proteins specifically bound the RV 3'(+)SL RNA that is required for the initiation of (-) strand RNA synthesis, it was important to identify such cellular RNA binding factors. A ~60-kDa protein was purified to near homogeneity from uninfected Vero 76 cytosolic lysates (Fig. 7.4A, lane 1).[35] Incubation of the purified protein with radiolabeled RV 3'(+)SL RNA in a UV crosslinking assay resulted in the labeling of the ~60-kDa protein (Fig. 7.4A, compare lanes 1 and 2), confirming that we had purified the authentic RNA binding protein of interest. Comparison of the amino acid sequence of five tryptic peptides derived from the 60-kDa protein showed that it had a 96% identity with human calreticulin (Fig. 7.4B). The identity of the simian calreticulin was further established by its specific immunoreactivity with antibodies raised against human calreticulin peptides.[35] Since we knew from our previous studies that the host-proteins binding to the 3'(+)SL RNA were highly dependent on their phosphorylation state, we determined the phosphorylation status of calreticulin in vivo. Uninfected and RV-infected Vero 76 cells were labeled with ^{32}P-orthophosphoric acid and the labeled cytosolic proteins were immunoprecipitated with calreticulin-specific antiserum. A major labeled protein of ~60-kDa was observed

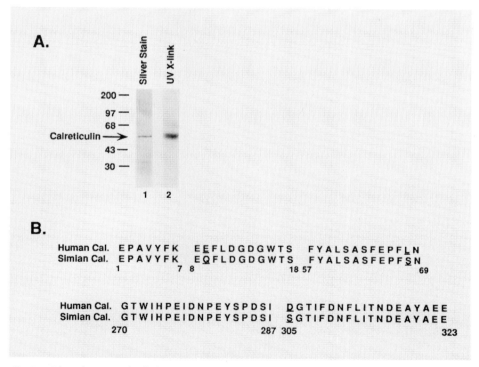

Fig. 7.4. Identification of cellular protein binding the RV 3'(+)SL RNA as calreticulin. A. Purified Vero 76 (simian) cellular protein (~60-kDa) is shown following silver staining (lane 1) and after incubation with radiolabeled RV 3'(+)SL RNA and UV crosslinking (lane 2). Only the ~60 kDa protein retains label from the RNA probe following UV crosslinking, confirming that it is the RNA binding protein of interest. B. Comparison of the amino acid (aa) sequence of five tryptic peptides derived from the purified ~60-kDa protein with cognate sequences in human calreticulin. Numbers on bottom represent aa numbers of the human sequence. Underlined amino acids indicate differences between the simian and human calreticulin sequences.

in both cell lysates (Fig. 7.5A), establishing that calreticulin is a phosphoprotein. However, there were two fold greater amounts of label associated with calreticulin in infected cell lysates, than in uninfected lysates without a concomitant change in steady state levels (Fig. 7.5A, lanes 2 and 3, compare 7.5B, lanes 1 and 2). This suggested that RV infection induces the hyperphosphorylation of calreticulin and conclusively demonstrated that we had identified the RV RNA binding protein as a phosphorylated form of simian calreticulin.[35]

IN VIVO ASSOCIATION OF CALRETICULIN WITH RV RNA

Under in vitro conditions, which often do not conform to the complex physiological conditions within the cell, purified cellular

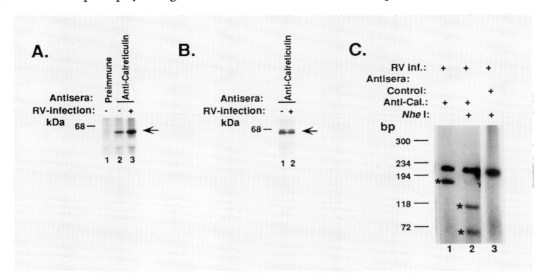

Fig. 7.5. Demonstration of calreticulin as a phosphoprotein and its association with 3'(+)SL RNA in vivo. A. Vero 76 cells were metabolically labeled with ^{32}P-orthophosphoric acid and cellular lysates were subjected to immunoprecipitation using a human calreticulin specific antibody. Products immunoprecipitated with pre-immune sera is shown in lane 1, while precipitation products from uninfected (lane 2) and RV infected lysates (lane 3) using anti-calreticulin sera are indicated by arrow. B. Equal amounts of labeled cellular proteins (described in A) from uninfected (lane 1) or RV infected (lane 2) cells were separated by SDS-PAGE and immunoblotted with anti-calreticulin antibodies. Arrow indicates the position of calreticulin. C. RV 3'(+)SL RNA complexed with calreticulin in RV infected Vero 76 cells was detected by exposing intact cells to UV light. Isolation of RNA-protein complexes by immunoprecipitation with indicated antisera, and isolation of RNA components is described in Singh et al.[35] RV RNA immunoprecipitated in this manner was detected by reverse transcription followed by polymerase chain reaction (RT-PCR) amplification. RNA products immunoprecipitated with anti-calreticulin sera: lane 1, a PCR product of 161 bp (*) amplified by RT-PCR; lane 2, 161 bp product is digested with Nhe I restriction enzyme which cleaves into 98 (*) and 63 (*) size fragments. Immunoprecipitations using control antisera yielded no RV specific 161 bp amplification product (lane 3).

proteins can bind to specific RNAs. However, demonstration of such association in vivo is critical before implicating biological functions to such an association. We demonstrated the in vivo association of calreticulin with the RV 3'(+)SL RNA by exposing intact RV-infected Vero 76 cells to UV light and immunoprecipitating RNP complexes present in cytolysates prepared from these cells using a calreticulin-specific antibody. The RV 3'(+)RNA present in the RNP complexes was then detected by reverse transcription followed by polymerase chain reaction (RT-PCR) amplification. An amplified product derived from the RV 3'(+) terminal RNA sequences could be distinguished from contaminating amplification products by a diagnostic *Nhe I* restriction enzyme cleavage site within the virus cDNA (Fig. 7.3C). The RV specific primers specifically amplify a ~161 bp DNA from RNA derived from the immunoprecipitated RNPs (Fig. 7.5C, lane 1). Digestion of RT-PCR products with *Nhe I* cleaves the 161 bp product into 98 and 63 bp products (Fig. 7.5C, lane 2). These studies clearly demonstrated that calreticulin in RV infected cells specifically interacts with the 3'(+)SL structure within the RV genome and we postulate that this binding contributes to RV replication.[35]

CALRETICULIN FUNCTIONS: FROM Ca^{2+} STORAGE TO VIRAL RNA BINDING PROTEIN

The diverse functions associated with calreticulin have emerged rapidly and many are presented in detail in accompanying chapters of this monograph. Calreticulin has three major putative structural domains (Chapter 2); a globular N-terminal domain, a proline-rich P-domain and an acidic C-terminal domain (Fig. 7.9).[36] The P- and C-domains contain the Ca^{2+} storage properties (Chapter 5).[36] Recently, it has been shown that calreticulin modulates the expression of hormonally regulated genes (Chapter 6), and has also been localized to other cellular organelles (Chapter 3 and 9), supporting its possible functional activity outside the endoplasmic reticulum.[37-39] The globular N-terminal domain was shown to have affinity for the cytoplasmic domain of the α-subunit of integrins and for a family of steroid receptors.[37-40] Recent studies suggest that the calreticulin-integrin interaction plays a crucial role in integrin mediated cell-ECM (extracellular matrix substrates) interactions.[40] As an iron-binding protein, calreticulin is present in duodenal mucosa and is implicated in iron uptake via a transferrin-independent pathway.[41,42] Calreticulin was also identified as a new rheumatic disease autoantigen that is intimately associated with the Ro/SS-A ribonucleoprotein complex (Chapter 8).[43] Results from our laboratory have confirmed this observation by showing that RNP complexes of calreticulin and the RV 3'(+)SL RNA can be immunoprecipitated by a subset of SSA and SS-A/SS-B type sera derived from RV-positive patients with autoimmune dysfunctions (Hofmann et al unpublished data). However, it remains to be seen whether sera from patients with RV-associated arthritis (one of the disease manifestations of chronic RV infection) contain antibodies which recognize calreticulin-RV RNA complexes. The prevalence of such reactivity could establish a connection between the calreticulin-RV RNA interaction and disease aspects emerging from persistent RV infections.

In addition to the above mentioned functions attributed to calreticulin, our laboratory has been the first to demonstrate that calreticulin is an RNA binding protein and that a phosphorylated form specifically binds RV RNA.[35,44] The newly discovered RNA binding function was further demonstrated in vitro using protein derived from a cDNA clone of human calreticulin fused with the maltose-binding protein (Cal-MBP) and expressed in *E. coli*.[35] This allowed careful functional analysis of the RNA-binding properties of calreticulin to be determined. Incubation of purified Cal-MBP with RV 3'(+) SL RNA resulted in no measurable RNA binding activity, which was not surprising, since we had previously established that phosphorylation was necessary for calreticulin in crude Vero cytolysates to bind the RV 3'(+)SL RNA.[32] Cal-MBP was then subjected to an in vitro phosphorylation reaction in the absence and presence of Vero cell cytolysates. Unexpectedly, we found that Cal-MBP was labeled with ^{32}P in the absence of cytolysates (Fig. 7.6A, lane 2). This raised the possibility that calreticulin may have autokinase activity. To confirm that this was indeed the case, we incubated Cal-MBP with a non-hydrolysable ATP analogue (^{35}S-ATP) and then separated the resulting complexes by 2-dimensional gel electrophoresis. The resulting gel was stained with coomassie blue and subsequently subjected to autoradiography. The autoradiographic signal co-migrated with the stained band of Cal-MBP, which suggested that phosphorylation of calreticulin in the reaction was not due to any contaminating kinase and that calreticulin is an autokinase (Singh et al, unpublished data). Similar kinase reactions with MBP alone showed no phosphorylation activity (Fig. 7.6A, lane 1). Phosphoamino acid analysis of recombinant calreticulin revealed that serine and threonine residues undergo autophosphorylation.[44] However, at present, we do not know the cellular protein substrates for the kinase activity of calreticulin, nor do we know if calreticulin is a substrate for other cellular kinases.

To establish that phosphorylated Cal-MBP binds to RV 3'(+)SL RNA, Cal-MBP and MBP were subjected to in vitro phosphorylation with unlabeled ATP and then incubated separately with the radiolabeled 3'(+)SL RNA. The resulting RNA mobility-shift gel showed that only the Cal-MBP fusion protein that was subjected to autophosphorylation bound the RV RNA (Fig. 7.6B, compare lane 2 with 4). In a similar experiment, MBP showed no interactions with the labeled RNA (Fig. 7.6B, lane 1). Treatment of the

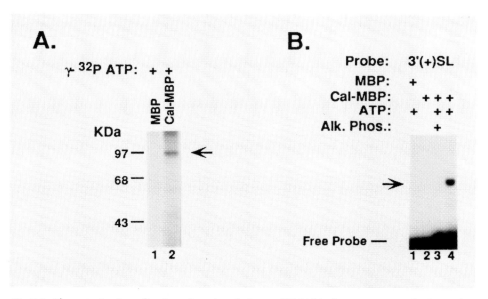

Fig. 7.6. Characterization of in vitro phosphorylation and RNA binding properties of calreticulin. Calreticulin was expressed in E. coli as a maltose binding fusion protein (Cal-MBP). In other experiments maltose binding protein (MBP) was expressed alone. A. Purified MBP or Cal-MBP fusion proteins were subjected to autophosphorylation reactions in the presence of γ-^{32}P ATP and products were separated by SDS-PAGE: MBP (lane 1), Cal-MBP (lane 2). The arrow indicates the position of labeled Cal-MBP. B. Cal-MBP or MBP alone were subjected to autophosphorylation reactions in the presence of unlabeled ATP, incubated with radiolabeled 3'(+)SL RNA and RNA-protein complexes were resolved in a non-denaturing polyacrylamide gels. The 3'(+)SL RNA was incubated with: MBP subjected to autophosphorylation conditions (lane 1); Cal-MBP untreated (lane 2); Cal-MBP subjected to autophosphorylation, followed by alkaline phosphatase treatment (lane 3); Cal-MBP subjected to autophosphorylation conditions (lane 4). Arrow indicates the position of the RNA-protein complex.

phosphorylated Cal-MBP with alkaline phosphatase prior to its incubation with RV RNA abrogated the binding of Cal-MBP (Fig. 7.6B, lane 3), providing evidence that autophosphorylation converts calreticulin into an RNA binding protein.

From such studies, it was obvious that calreticulin is converted into a RV RNA binding protein by an autokinase activity. These studies, however, did not reveal regions within calreticulin responsible for RNA binding and autokinase activities. To define the regions of calreticulin conferring autophosphorylation and RNA binding activities, the putative N-, P- and C-domains of human calreticulin were expressed as MBP fusion proteins (Fig. 7.7).[44] Autophosphorylation of recombinant proteins showed that only intact calreticulin or the N-domain proteins were capable of either autophosphorylation or RV RNA binding (Fig. 7.7). However, we

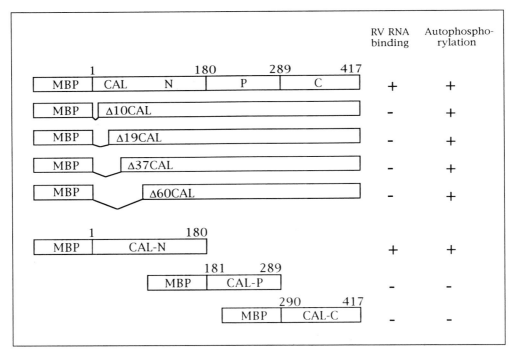

Fig. 7.7. Schematic representation of full-length, individual domains and truncated portions of human calreticulin expressed in E. coli as MBP-fusion proteins. Fusion proteins are represented as boxes. MBP denotes maltose binding protein and Cal-N-, P- and C- represent individual polypeptide domains determined in the human calreticulin sequence by its homology with rabbit calreticulin.[36] Numbers on top of each box denote the amino acid numbers taken from mature human calreticulin.[59] The RNA binding and phosphorylation activities were measured as indicated in the legend to Figure 7.6. On the right, the performance of each fusion protein in RNA binding and phosphorylation activities is indicated by positive (+) or negative (-) symbols.

can not rule out whether the lack of phosphorus labeling of the P and C domains of calreticulin is due to the absence of the N-domain. In other experiments, deletions were introduced into the N-domain of recombinant calreticulin to further localize functional regions.[44] Deletions of up to 60 N-terminal amino acids did not alter the ability of the fusion proteins to autophosphorylate, whereas RNA binding activity was abolished by deletion of as few as the first 10 amino acids (Fig. 7.7). Therefore, one could conclude from such studies that the RNA binding and phosphorylation domains of calreticulin are distinct, but at the same time, both domains must be present to confer the RNA binding activity.[44]

RELATIONSHIP OF CALRETICULIN TO OTHER KNOWN RNA BINDING PROTEINS

It is commonly thought that for RNA binding to occur, proteins must contain certain conserved RNA recognition motifs (RRM).[45] However, no RRM motifs were identified in the deduced amino acid sequence of calreticulin; nevertheless, calreticulin specifically binds RV RNA. Since it was determined that the N-terminal 10 amino acids of calreticulin are essential for the RNA binding activity, it was logical to seek to identify any putative functional resemblance between this sequence and other RNA binding proteins. Such an analysis revealed the presence of a pentameric motif (A-V-Y-F-K) in RNA binding proteins, including calreticulin, outside their known RRM motifs (Table 7.1). Further, a similar motif (N-V-Y-I-K) is also present in the RNP2 repeat sequence of the poly(A)-binding protein of human and *Xenopus laevis*[46,47] as well as within RNP1 motif (F-V-I-F-K) of human U1 small nuclear RNP A1 and U2 snRNP B"1.[48] Interestingly, RV coat protein[49] which interacts with RV RNA in the viral RNA packaging, also contains a AVFYR motif (Table 7.1). Thus, it seems that the RRM motifs alone may not contain sufficient information for certain proteins to function in RNA binding. However, the presence of amino acid sequences contributing to RNA binding, flanking the RRMs, suggests that the ancillary motifs may function in the maintenance of protein structure, enabling proteins to make correct contacts with their target RNAs.

Despite the absence of a consensus RRM, the phosphorylated form of calreticulin exhibits a strong RV RNA-binding activity (Figs. 7.3-7.6). It is known that RNA binding proteins, such as glyceraldehyde-3-phosphate dehydrogenase (GAPDH) and the cytoplasmic aconitase, which constitutes the iron responsive element binding protein (IRE-BP), also lack RRMs. The RNA-binding activities of these two proteins are regulated by the presence or absence of their respective co-factors, NAD^+ and iron-sulfur cluster.[50, 51] Since phosphorylation of calreticulin is crucial for RV RNA-binding, we believe that in the cell, phosphorylation regulates and recruits calreticulin for RNA-binding. This is evident by the observation that while calreticulin is a moderately abundant protein in Vero 76 cells, only a fraction of it is phosphorylated upon RV infection (Fig. 7.5, compare panels A and B). Post-translational modifications such as phosphorylation are known to have regulatory functions that affect the properties of a wide range of proteins. For example, in human hnRNP protein A1, phosphorylation

Table 7.1 Amino acid comparison of putative RNA-binding motif of calreticulin with other RNA-binding protein sequences

Protein	Start	Sequence						End
Human:								
1. Calreticulin N-terminus	3	A	V	Y	F	K	E	8
2. La	112	S	V	Y	I	K	G	117
3. U1 SnRNP 70K	134	M	V	Y	S	K	R	139
4. U2 SnRNP-B"#1 (RNP1)	53	F	V	I	F	K	E	58
5. U1 SnRNP-A #1 (RNP1)	56	F	V	I	F	K	E	61
6. Poly(A) BP #1	75	D	V	-	I	K	G	79
7. Poly(A) BP #3 (RNP2)	192	N	V	Y	I	K	N	197
8. hnRNP K	56	A	V	I	G	K	G	61
9. SF2 a)	35	D	V	F	Y	K	Y	40
b)	71	A	V	Y	G	R	D	76
Xenopus laevis :								
10. hnRNP K	53	A	V	I	G	K	G	58
11. Poly(A) BP (RNP2)	192	N	V	Y	I	K	N	197
12. RV Coat protein	165	A	V	F	Y	R	V	170
Putative Consensus Sequence		A	V	Y	X	K	X	
		X		I		R		
				F				

1. McCauliffe et al, 1990
2. Query et al, 1989)
3-7 & 9. Krainer et al, 1991
8 & 10. Siomi et al, 1993
11. Nietfeld et al, 1990
12. Dominguez et al, 1990

by cAMP-dependent protein kinase suppresses the capacity of protein A1 to promote strand annealing in vitro, without altering its ability to bind to nucleic acid.[52]

The lack of typical RRMs[53] among RNA binding proteins such as calreticulin,[35] IRE-BP,[50] GAPDH,[51] tRNA synthetases[54] and the HIV tat protein,[55] leads us to speculate that there are several types of RNA-binding proteins within most cells. For example, some proteins that contain RRM motifs are dedicated for general RNA metabolism, including the splicing, stability and translation of mRNAs. Whereas other proteins, that lack conserved RRMs, have primary "house keeping" functions within the cell, e.g. participating in energy metabolism or Ca^{2+} storage. In the latter group, sequence motifs other than RRMs have been recruited to function as RNA binding domains. Further, post-translational modifications of such proteins may also be necessary to induce conformational changes, juxtaposing the necessary residues in a binding pocket. Members of this multi-functional group of RNA binding proteins, including calreticulin, GAPDH and the IRE-BP, may bind specific RNAs and thus regulate discrete metabolic events within the cell.

PUTATIVE CONTRIBUTIONS OF CALRETICULIN IN RV REPLICATION

As discussed earlier in this chapter, RV replication is severely limited by inhibition of host protein expression during the initial hours of infection (Fig. 7.2). This result suggested that host factors for minimal replication are pre-existent in uninfected cells, but RV infection induces the accumulation or modification of newly translated host-encoded proteins which stimulate further replication. We have shown that RV infection induces the hyperphosphorylation of calreticulin, as evidenced by the slower migrating forms (~63- and 68-kDa) of proteins binding the RV RNA from infected cytolysates (Fig. 7.3B)[32] and reacting with calreticulin specific sera (Fig. 7.5A). However, steady state levels of major calreticulin forms show little change in response to RV infection (Fig. 7.5B). It is also known that the number of binding sites for the RV 3'(+)SL increases from ~2100 sites in uninfected Vero cells to ~15,000 sites in RV infected cells.[32] This increase in binding activity temporally corresponds to the initiation of detectable RV (-) strand RNA synthesis.[32] Increases in the specific binding activity of calreticulin in RV infected cells can be attributed to the induction of hyperphosphorylation of newly translated calreticulin.[32] Further, this hyperphosphorylation may even induce the redistribution of newly translated calreticulin, from primarily endoplasmic reticulum targeting, to retention in the cytoplasm. In this model, we propose that the number of calreticulin molecules in a cell is not the most important variable, but the nature and competency of the calreticulin molecules distributed in the cytosol is essential.

The fact that minimal levels of RV replication can be observed in cells pre-treated with Actinomycin D (or treatment 2 or 4 hours post infection; Fig. 7.2) is consistent with the observation that low levels of appropriately modified calreticulin exist in Vero 76 cells at all times (Fig. 7.3A, lane 1). However, calreticulin was not similarly modified in some other cell lines. The RV 3'(+)SL RNA binding activities present in cell lines derived from a variety of lineages was tested by UV crosslinking analysis with the resulting products resolved by SDS-PAGE and blotted to filters (Fig. 7.8).

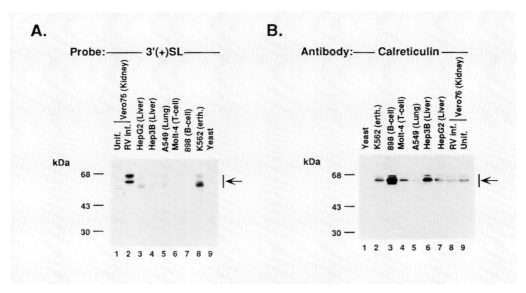

Fig. 7.8. The presence of calreticulin and its ability to bind the RV 3'(+)SL RNA in cytolysates derived from different cell types. A. Radiolabeled RV 3'(+)SL RNA was incubated with cytolysates from several cell lines (source indicated above each lane). Following treatment with UV light, RNA-binding proteins were analyzed by SDS-PAGE and blotted onto nitrocellulose paper. Proteins labeled due to their association with the RV 3'(+)SL RNA were visualized by autoradiography and observed in each cell type with the exception of B cell and T cell lines and yeast. B. Following identification of RNA binding activities, the blot of UV crosslinking products in A. was subjected to Western blot analysis using antibodies raised against human calreticulin. Arrow indicates the position of the calreticulin which, in each case, co-migrates with labeled proteins in A.

The same filter was first exposed for autoradiography and then subjected to Western blotting using calreticulin specific anti-sera. Several cell lines derived from liver, lung or erythrocytes contained levels of calreticulin and binding activities similar to that observed in Vero 76 cells (Fig. 7.8A, lanes 1-5, 8; Fig. 7.8B, lanes 2, 5-9). Of particular interest is the very strong binding pattern observed in erythrocyte cells (Fig. 7.8A, lane 8). In contrast, copious quantities of calreticulin are found in B and T cell lines, but no RNA binding activity was observed (Fig. 7.8A, lanes 6-7; Fig. 7.8B, lanes 3-4), suggesting that the endogenous calreticulin in these cultured cells is not properly modified for RNA binding. Initial RV infections are thought to be in monocytes, although RV infections of B- and T-cells have been reported.[20] The lack of calreticulin-mediated RNA binding in B and T cells may present a conflict with our contention for the involvement of calreticulin in RV replication. However, interactions between infected monocytes and B- and T cells is necessary for the induction of humoral and cellular immune responses to clear RV infections. The interactions between infected cells and B and T cells may induce the hyperphosphorylation of calreticulin within these immune system cells, thus creating a pool of RNA-binding competent proteins to support RV infections. These results further confirm our contention that the nature of modifications to calreticulin, rather than its abundance, is the determining factor for RNA binding. Finally, treatment of RV infected Vero cells with AMD, 8 hours following RV infection, allows a near normal replication pattern (Fig. 7.2) indicating that by this time a threshold amount of modified calreticulin has accumulated to support RNA replication. These results taken together suggest that RV infection induces the production of a diverse pool of calreticulin proteins which can serve in the replication of RV RNA.

FUTURE PERSPECTIVES

The phosphorylation status of calreticulin is critical for it to bind the RV 3'(+)SL RNA; however, this association has hitherto only been implicated in RV replication. A key question remaining to be answered is whether binding of calreticulin to the RV 3'(+)SL regulates RV replication. This hypothesis can be tested by modulating the expression of calreticulin in Vero cells followed by analysis of the effects of such alterations on RV replication. In addition, we know that hyperphosphorylation of calreticulin is increased upon RV infection, coinciding with the detection of RV (-) strand RNA synthesis, therefore, it is important to elucidate the pathway by which calreticulin is phosphorylated in RV infected Vero cells. Studies are in progress to determine the mechanism by which modifications of calreticulin are induced upon RV infection. Further, the regulation of the autokinase activity of calreticulin in both uninfected and RV infected Vero cells as well as the activities of other cellular kinases on calreticulin need to be studied.

If calreticulin plays a significant role in RV replication, it will be important to resolve the context in which calreticulin exerts its influence; does calreticulin act independently or in concert with virus-encoded nonstructural proteins, thus promoting initiation of RNA synthesis at the 3' terminus of the RV RNA. Studies are in progress to evaluate the potential interactions of calreticulin with RV non-structural proteins both in vitro and in vivo. If interactions between calreticulin and RV nonstructural proteins are described, the contributions to RV replication can be studied by altering protein-protein interactions.

A productive RV infection affects overall cellular metabolism which can be observed in the growth arrest of fetal tissues infected with RV.[21] Such slowed mitotic rates have been implicated as the cause of the teratogenic effects of RV infection on fetal development.[21]

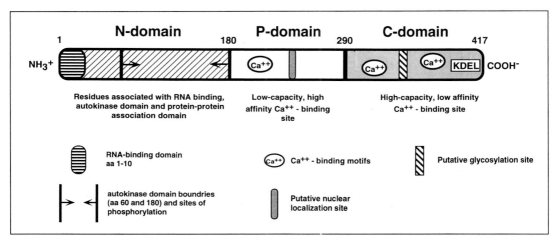

Fig. 7.9. Schematic representation of human calreticulin,[59] with functional domains denoted with various symbols as indicated in legend. New functional domains elucidated by our laboratory and described in this chapter include the residues contributing to RNA binding (N-terminal residues 1-10) and autokinase (N-terminal residues 60-180) activities. Amino acid (aa) numbers demarking distinct domains are indicated above diagram.

Similarly, RV infections of cultured human diploid fibroblasts resulted in mitotic arrest.[56] Indeed, we have previously observed that growth arrested Vero 76 cells are much more susceptible to RV infections and have significantly higher RNA binding activity of calreticulin.[32] Further, preliminary studies in our laboratory with cell cycle regulation in RV infected cells suggest that a significant population of infected cells are arrested at G2/M phase (Singh et al, unpublished data). In similar experiments cell cycle dependent phosphorylation of calreticulin is also altered. Therefore, studying the molecular mechanisms supporting both the cell cycle dependent phosphorylation of calreticulin and RV infections and the manner in which they compliment each other will be important for understanding the basis of RV pathogenesis.

CONCLUSIONS

In this chapter we have described the identification and characterization of a host protein, the phosphorylated form of calreticulin, that specifically binds the RV 3'(+)SL *cis*-acting element in vitro as well as in vivo, during RV infection. For the first time, calreticulin has been shown to be an RNA binding protein, although it also possesses numerous other activities, some of which are described in other portions of this monograph. Both the RNA binding and autokinase activities of calreticulin are present in the putative globular N-domain. It was also demonstrated that only phosphorylated calreticulin functions as an RNA binding protein and that calreticulin possesses a serine/threonine autokinase activity. We have also provided evidence on how initial events during the RV replication cycle induce changes in cellular metabolism rendering the cell more permissive for virus multiplication. Chief among these metabolic alterations is the induction of hyper-phosphorylation of newly translated calreticulin, which dramatically increases its RV RNA binding activity. Although the implications of the binding of calreticulin to a *cis*-acting element of the RV RNA are only speculative, we believe that continued study of RV RNA-calreticulin interaction will provide new understanding of RV pathogenesis. The implications of such interactions may provide insight into cellular abnormalities associated with RV infection, including the development of persistent RV infections, teratogenic effects of RV infections on developing tissues and autoimmune-like symptoms accompanying RV-associated arthritis.

ACKNOWLEDGMENTS

We are grateful to Dr R. Sontheimer for the generous gift of calreticulin antibodies and human calreticulin cDNA. We thank Drs. Tosato, Egan and Duncan for their critical review. We appreciate Dr. G. Tosato for constant support and encouragment.

REFERENCES

1. Hershey HV, Taylor MW. Strategy of replication of the viral genome. In: Bercoff RP, ed. The molecular basis of viral replication. NATO ASI Series 1987; 47-98.

2. Mendelshon CL, Wimmer E, Racaniello VR. Cellular receptor for poliovirus: molecular cloning, nucleotide sequence, and expression of a new member of the immunoglobulin superfamily. Cell 1989; 56:855-865.

3. Doring RE, Marcil A, Chopra A et al. The human CD46 molecule is a receptor for measles virus (Edmonton strain). Cell 1993; 75:295-305.

4. Strauss JH, Wang K-S, Schmaljohn AL et al. Host-cell receptors for sindbis virus. Arch Virol 1994; 9:473-484.

5. Andino R, Rieckhof GE, Achacoso PL et al. Poliovirus RNA synthesis utilizes an RNA complex formed around the 5' end of viral RNA. EMBO J 1993; 12:3587-3598.

6. Pogue GP, Huntley CC, Hall TC. Common replication strategies emerging from the study of diverse groups of positive-strand RNA viruses. Arch Virol 1994; 9:181-194.

7. Nakhasi HL, Singh NK, Pogue GP et al. Identification and characterization of host factor interactions with cis-acting elements of rubella virus RNA. Arch Virol 1994; 9:255-267.

8. Porter A. Picornavirus nonstructural proteins: emerging roles in virus replication and inhibition of host cell functions. J Virol 1993; 67:6917-6921.

9. Strauss JH, Kuhn RJ, Niesters HGM et al. Functions of the 5'-terminal and 3'-terminal sequences of the sindbis virus genome in replication. In: Brinton MA, Heinz FX, ed. New aspects of positive-strand RNA viruses. Am Soc Microbiol Washington DC 1990; 61-66.

10. Biebricker C K, Eigen M. Kinetics of RNA replication by Qβ replicase. In: Domingo E, Holland JJ, Ahlquist P, ed. RNA Genetics: RNA-directed virus rerplication. CRC Press, Boca Raton, Florida. 1988; 1-18.

11. Afzal MA, Elliott GD, Rima BK et al. Virus and host cell-dependent variation in transcription of the mumps virus genome. J Gen Virol 1990; 71:615-619.

12. De BP, Galinski MS, Banerjee A K. Human parainfluenza virus type 3 transcription in vitro: role of the cellular actin in mRNA synthesis. J Virol 1990; 64:1135-1142.

13. Hill AM, Harmon SH, Summers DF. Stimulation of vesicular stomatitis virus in vitro RNA synthesis by microtubule-associated proteins. Proc Natl Acad Sci USA 1986; 83:5410-5313.

14. Moyer SA, Baker SC, Horikami M. Host cell proteins required for measles virus reproduction. J Gen Virol 1990; 71:775-783.

15. Meerovitch K, Svitkin YV, Lee HS et al. La autoantigen enhances and corrects aberrant translation of poliovirus RNA in reticulocyte lysate. J Virol 1993; 67:3798-3807.

16. Chang Y-N, Kenan DJ, Keene JD et al. Direct interaction between autoantigen La and human immunodeficiency virus leader RNA. J Virol 1994; 68:7008-7020.

17. Svitkin YV, Pause A, Sonenberg N. La autoantigen alleviates translational repression by the 5' leader sequence of the human immunodeficiency virus type 1 mRNA. J Virol 1994; 68:7001-7007.

18. Pogue GP, Cao X-Q, Singh NK et al. 5' sequences of rubella virus RNA stimulate translation of chimeric RNA and specifically interact with two host-encoded proteins. J Virol 1993; 67:7106-7117.

19. International committee on taxonomy of viruses: classification and nomenclature of viruses. Arch Virol 1991; 2:219.

20. Wolinsky JS, Rubella. In: Fields BN, Knipe DM. ed. Virology, Raven, New York 1990; 1:815-838.

21. Naeye RL, Blanc W. Pathogenesis of congenital rubella. J Amer Med Assoc 1965; 194:1277.

22. Spruance SL, Smith CB. Joint complications associated with derivatives of HPV-77 rubella virus vaccine. Am J Dis Child 1971; 122:105-111.

23. Howson CP, Katz M, Johnston RB et al. Chronic Arthritis after rubella vaccination. Clin Infect Dis 1992; 15:307-312.

24. Adverse effects of pertussis and rubella vaccines. In: Howson CP, Howe CJ, Fineberg HV, ed. A report of the committee to review the adverse consequences of pertussis and rubella vaccines. Division of health promotion and disease prevention. Natl Acad Press 1991; 187-197.

25. Frey TK. Molecular biology of rubella virus. Adv Virus Res 1994; 44:69-160.

26. Forng R-Y, Frey TK. Identification of the rubella virus nonstructural proteins. Virol 1995; 206:843-853.

27. Oker-Blom C, Ulmenen I, Kaanianen L et al. Rubella virus 40S genome RNA specifies a 24S subgenomic mRNA that codes for a precursor to structural proteins. J Virol 1984; 49:403-408.

28. Nakhasi HL, Zheng D, Hewlett IK et al. Rubella virus replication: effect of interferons and actinomycin D. Virus Res 1988; 10:1-15.

29. Sawicki DL, Sawicki SG. Short-lived minus-strand polymerase for Semliki forest virus. J Virol 1980; 34:108-118.

30. Strauss EG, Strauss JH. Structure and replication of the alphavirus genome. In: Schlesinger S, Schlesinger M J. ed. The Togaviridae and Flaviviridae. Plenum publishing Corp. 1986; 35-90.

31. Levis R, Weiss BG, Tsiang M et al. Deletion mapping of Sindbis virus DI RNAs derived from cDNAs defines the sequences essential for replication and packaging. Cell 1986; 44:137-145.

32. Nakhasi HL, Rouault TA, Haile DJ et al. Specific high-affinity binding of host cell proteins to the 3' region of rubella virus RNA. New Biol 1990; 2:255-264.

33. Chattopadhya D, Banerjee AK. Phosphorylation within a specific domain of the phosphoprotein of vesicular stomatitis virus regulates transcription in vitro. Cell 1987; 49:407-414.

34. Ransome LJ, Dasgupta A. Multiple isoelectric forms of poliovirus RNA-dependent RNA polymerase: evidence for phosphorylation. J Virol 1989; 63:4563-4568.

35. Singh NK, Atreya CD, Nakhasi HL. Identification of calreticulin as rubella virus RNA-binding protein. Proc Natl Acad Sci USA 1994; 91:12770-12774.

36. Michalak R, Milner RE, Burns K et al. Calreticulin. Biochem J 1992; 285:681-692.

37. Burns KB, Duggan EA, Atkinson KS et al. 1994. Modulation of gene expression by calreticulin binding to the glucocotricoid receptor. Nature 367:476-480.

38. Dedhar S, Rennie P, Shago M et al. Inhibition of nuclear hormone receptor activity by calreticulin. Nature 1994; 367:480-483.

39. Dedhar S. Novel functions for calreticulin: interaction with integrins and modulation of gene expression? TIBS 1994; 19:269-271.

40. Leung-Hagesteinjn CY, Milankov K, Michalak M et al. Cell attachment matrix substrates is inhibited upon downregulation of expression of calreticulin, an intracellular integrin α-subunit-binding protein. J Cell Sci 1994; 107:589-600.

41. Conrad ME, Umbreit JN, Moore EG et al. A newly identified iron binding protein in duodenal mucosa of rats: Purification and characterization of mobilferrin. J Biol Chem 1990; 265:5273-5279.

42. Conrad ME, Umbreit JN. A concise review of iron absorption: the mucin-mobilferrin-integrin pathway. A competitive pathway for metal absorption. Am J Hematol 1993; 42:67-73.

43. Sontheimer RD, Lieu T-S, Capra JD. Calreticulin: the diverse functional repertoire of a new human autoantigen. The Immunologist 1993; 5:155-160.

44. Atreya CD, Singh NK, Nakhasi HL. The RNA binding activity of human calreticulin is localized to the N-terminal domain. JVirol 1995; 69:3848-3851.

45. Burd CG, Dreyfuss G. Conserved structures and diversity of functions of RNA-binding proteins. Science 1994; 265:615-621.

46. Grange T, Martin C, Oddos J et al. Human mRNA poly adenylate binding protein: evolutionary conservation of a nucleic acid binding motif. Nucl Acids Res 1987; 15:4771-4787.

47. Nietfeld W, Mentzel H, Pieler T. The *Xenopus laevis* poly(A) binding protein is composed of multiple functionally independent RNA binding domains. EMBO J 1990; 9:3699-3705.

48. Krainer AR, Mayeda A, Kozak D et al. Functional expression of cloned human splicing factor SF2: homology to RNA-binding proteins, U1 70K, and Drosophila splicing regulators. Cell 1991; 66:383-394.

49. Zheng D, Dickens L, Liu T-Y et al. Nucleotide sequence of the 24S subgenomic messenger RNA of a vaccine strain (HPV 77) of rubella virus: comparison with a wild type strain (M33). Gene 1989; 82:343-349.

50. Klausner RD, Rouault TA, Harford JB. Regulating the fate of mRNA: the control of cellular iron metabolism. Cell 1993; 72:19-28.

51. Singh R, Green MR. Sequence-specific binding of transfer RNA by glyceraldehyde-3-phosphate dehydrogenase. Science 1993; 259:365-368.

52. Cobianchi F, Calvio C, Stoppini M et al. Phosphorylation of human hnRNP protein A1 abrogates in vitro strand annealing activity. Nucl Acids Res 1993; 21:949-955.

53. Kenan DJ, Query CC, Keene JD. RNA recognition: towards identifying determinants of specificity. TIBS 1991; 16:214-220.

54. Rould MA, Perona JJ, Soll DD et al. Structure of *E. coli* glutaminyl-tRNA synthetase complexed with tRNA^{Gln} and ATP at 2.8 Å resolution. Science 1989; 246:1135-1142.

55. Cordingley MG, LaFamina RL, Callahan PL et al. Sequence-specific interaction of Tat protein and Tat peptides with the transactivation-repressive sequence element of human immunodeficiency virus type 1 in vitro. Proc Natl Acad Sci USA 1990; 87:8985-8989.

56. Plotkin SA, Vaheri A. Human fibroblasts infected with rubella virus produce a growth inhibitor. Science 1967; 156:659-661.

57. Query CC, Bentley RC, Keene JD. A common RNA recognition motif identified within a defined U1 RNA binding domain of the 70K U1 snRNP protein. Cell 1989; 57:89-101.

58. Siomi H, Matunis MJ, Michael WM et al. The pre-mRNA binding K protein contains a novel evolutionarily conserved motif. Nucl Acids Res 1993; 21:1193-1198.

59. McCauliffe DP, Zappi E, Lui TS et al. A human Ro/SS-A autoantigen is the homologue of calreticulin and is highly homologous with onchoceral RAL-1 antigen and an aplysia "memory molecule". J Clin Invest 1990; 86:332-335.

CHAPTER 8

CALRETICULIN AND AUTOIMMUNITY

Richard D. Sontheimer, Tho Q. Nguyen, Shih-Tsung Cheng, Tsu-San Lieu and J. Donald Capra

INTRODUCTION

The human calreticulin amino acid sequence has been shown to be associated with the immune response in several ways. In addition, calreticulin is now widely accepted to be the target of autoantibody production in several autoimmune diseases including systemic lupus erythematosus (SLE). In this review, we have attempted to provide some perspective upon the relationship that exists between calreticulin and the autoimmune response, focusing especially upon the confusing and highly-debated relationship that exists between calreticulin and the Ro/SS-A autoantigenic ribonucleoprotein (RNP). Space considerations do not allow a comprehensive review of all issues in this area. Additional discussion of the autoimmune aspects of calreticulin can be found in other recent publications.[1-3]

CALRETICULIN AND THE IMMUNE RESPONSE

Several observations suggest that calreticulin can be the target of protective immune responses. B50, the murine B16 melanoma tumor antigen that is also widely expressed on many types of rapidly proliferating cell lines, has been shown to be highly homologous to calreticulin.[4,5] The homologue of calreticulin that is expressed by the filarial parasite, *Onchocercai volvulus*, has been shown to be an immunodominant antigen in human onchocerciasis.[6,7] Similar observations have been made in another human parasitic disease, shistosomiasis. Shistosomiasis patient sera have been shown to contain antibodies that react with the *Schistosoma mansoni* form of calreticulin.[8]

CALRETICULIN AND THE AUTOIMMUNE RESPONSE ASSOCIATED WITH RHEUMATIC DISEASES

ORIGINAL DESCRIPTION OF CALRETICULIN AS A RHEUMATIC DISEASE-ASSOCIATED AUTOANTIGEN

A number of human rheumatic disease syndromes are characterized by the production of circulating autoantibodies that bind to RNP particles that are normally present in nucleated cells. These particles usually consist of multiple polypeptides associated with a single type of small RNA molecule. Ro/SS-A autoantibodies target one of these RNP particles, the cytoplasmic hYRNA RNP, and are characteristic of patients with SLE, subacute cutaneous LE, neonatal LE/ congenital heart block and Sjögren's syndrome (data reviewed in ref. 9). Much effort has been directed over the past 15 years toward characterizing the molecular constituents of the various RNP particles including hYRNA RNP with the hope that clues would be identified that might lead to the source of the autoimmune responses that are directed toward these particles. Studies from a number of labs have indicated that the Ro/SS-A RNP is quite complex, consisting of at least four antigenically distinct polypeptides between 52,000 and 60,000 in molecular weight that are associated with a unique class of small, uridine-rich, cytoplasmic RNA molecules known as the hYRNAs (data reviewed in ref. 10). In addition, the La/SS-B polypeptide also transiently associates with Ro/SS-A RNP particles.

In 1984 while working in Dr. Eng Tan's lab at the University of Colorado, Dr. Tsu-San Lieu developed for the first time an exclusively biochemical protocol for purifying a protein from human Wil-2 cells (the cell line in which the SS-A and SS-B autoantigens were originally identified) that migrated at 60-kDa in SDS-PAGE and reacted specifically with Ro/SS-A autoimmune sera in counterimmunoelectrophoresis (CIE).[11] Prior to that time, the 60-kDa Ro/SS-A polypeptide had been isolated only by immunoaffinity purification using patient sera. Because of its specific reactivity with anti-Ro/SS-A sera, its apparent molecular weight of 60,000, and a high 260:280 UV absorbance ratio suggesting the presence of associated nucleic acid, this protein was felt to represent the 60-kDa polypeptide component of the Ro/SS-A RNP particle.

After joining our lab in Dallas in 1985, Dr. Lieu's conclusions were further supported by the demonstration that his presumptive 60-kDa Ro/SS-A protein also reacted specifically with monospecific Ro/SS-A sera from our subacute cutaneous LE and Sjögren's syndrome patients when assayed under nondenaturing conditions

Fig. 8.1. Two dimensional gel (2D gel) analysis of the anti-Ro/SS-A autoantibody-reactive calreticulin fraction purified biochemically from human Wil-2 cells. Native Wil-2 cell calreticulin was purified by the procedure described in Table 1 with the modification that Sephacryl 300 column chromatography was used instead of native PAGE as the final purification step in this protocol to obtain higher yields. The purified calreticulin preparation was then run on high resolution 2-D gels. The sample was first separated by charge difference on pH 3-10 ampholine in a 5.5% polyacrylamide gel and then size-fractionated in the second dimension on a 12.5% SDS-PAGE gel. Isoelectric focusing was performed in the first dimension in 5.5% T, 2.6% C polyacrylamide containing 1% carrier ampholytes, pH 3-10 (Pharmacia). The upper chamber contained 0.5% ethanolamine and the lower chamber contained 0.05% sulfuric acid as electrolytes. The isoelectric focusing was carried at 4°C for 4 hours with final voltage of 600 V using an LKB 2197 power supply. Electrophoretic separation was performed in the second dimension in 12.5% T, 2.6% C polyacrylamide gel that contained 0.1% SDS, pH 8.8 with 3% stacking gel. The SDS-PAGE electrophoresis was considered complete when the bromophenol blue dye front was within 1 cm of the bottom of the gel. The gel was stained with 0.2% commassie brilliant blue. Commassie blue staining detected only a single acidic protein consistent in size and charge with calreticulin. These findings argue that the purified human Wil-2 cell calreticulin antigenic fractions that were used in our earlier studies were not contaminated with the more basic 60-kDa Ro/SS-A protein.

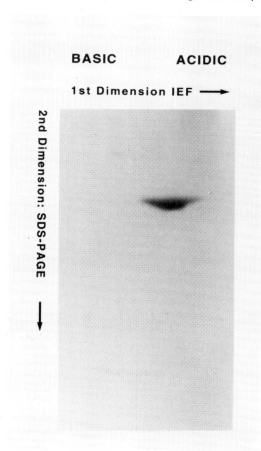

BASIC   **ACIDIC**

1st Dimension IEF ⟶

2nd Dimension: SDS-PAGE

Table 8.1. Differential reactivity of anti-Ro/SS-A autoimmune sera with native human calreticulin[1] under various assay conditions

Patient groups	# Positive/# Tested (% Positive)		
	CIE	ELISA[2]	Western blot[3]
SCLE:			
anti-Ro (+)	28/28 (100%)	27/28 (96%)	24/28 (86%)
anti-Ro (-)	0/10 (0%)	2/10 (20%)	0/2 (0%)
Drug-Induced SCLE	7/7 (100%)	6/7 (86%)	4/7 (57%)
Sjögren's Syndrome:			
anti-Ro (+)	16/16 (100%)	15/16 (94%)	10/16 (62%)
anti-Ro (-)	0/10 (0%)	Not done	1/10 (10%)
Mothers of infants with neonatal LE	9/9 (100%)	9/9 (100%)	6/9 (67%)
Disease controls	0/15 (0%)	3/15 (20%)	1/15 (7%)
Normal controls	0/10 (0%)	—	0/10 (0%)

[1]Native calreticulin was isolated from extracts of an Epstein-Barr virus transformed human B-lymphoblastoid cell line (Wil-2) by a procedure that has been previously described.[7,12] Briefly, cells were grown in Eagle's medium supplemented with 2 mM glutamine, sodium pyruvate, nonessential amino acids, 10% fetal calf serum, penicillin 10,000 U/ml, and streptomycin (10 mg/ml). The cells were centrifuged at 35 x g for 12 minutes and washed with phosphate buffered saline (PBS) three times. Approximately 40 ml of packed cells were then mixed with the same volume of PBS containing 1 mM PMSF. The suspension was sonicated on ice with ten 15-second pulses using a Heat System Sonicator at a setting of 9. The sonicate was then centrifuged at 12,100 x g for 1 h and the supernatant subjected to ammonium sulfate precipitation. The 33-80% ammonium sulfate fractions were dialyzed against 24 mM borate buffer, pH 7.6, and then applied to a polybuffer ion exchange column and eluted with a stepwise NaCl gradient at 4°C. Ro/SS-A antigenic activity was eluted from the column with 0.5 M and 1 M NaCl, concentrated, and immediately dialyzed in phosphate buffered saline pH 7.4. The 0.5-1.0 M NaCl fractions were further purified by preparative native PAGE. Ro/SS-A antigenic activity was then eluted from gel slices. The 260:280 absorbance ratio suggests that purified calreticulin is still associated with nucleic acid at this stage of purification. The presence of Ro/SS-A antigenic activity was monitored throughout this purification procedure by CIE against monospecific anti-Ro/SS-A sera that produce a line of identity with the CDC anti-Ro/SS-A reference serum, AF-CDC7 obtained from the CDC in Atlanta, Georgia.

[2]ELISA binding levels greater than two standard deviations above the mean of 100 normal blood bank control sera were considered positive.

[3]Western blot was carried out according to the method of Tobwin.[64] Proteins were electroblotted from SDS-PAGE gels onto nitrocellulose membrane at constant current (0.3 amps) for 3 hours. The membranes were first incubated with 1% bovine serum albumin in phosphate buffer-Tween solution for 1 hour at room temperature. After washing three times with PBS-Tween the membranes were incubated with antisera to rabbit skeletal muscle calreticulin (1:400) or autoimmune patient sera (1:100) for 2 hours. They were then washed for 15 minutes with PBS- Tween three times. This was followed by incubation with peroxidase conjugated swine anti-goat IgG (1:2000) or goat anti-human IgG (1:2000) respectively for 2 hours at room temperature and washed in a similar manner. The color was developed by reacting the membrane with 3.3 diaminobenzidine (20 mg/100 ml) in 50 mM Tris pH 7.5 with 1/10,000 volume of 30% H_2O_2.

such as CIE; however, this protein was found to be less reactive under the denaturing conditions of Western blot.[12-14] These differences are illustrated in the previously unpublished data presented in Table 8.1. Two dimensional gel (Fig. 8.1) and immunoblot (Fig. 8.2) studies subsequently confirmed that fractions containing this fully-purified Wil-2 cell protein were not contaminated with the 52- or 60-kDa Ro/SS-A polypeptides that had been discovered by other groups at about this same time.[15-17] The observation that a Ro/SS-A precipitate contains a Ca^{2+} binding protein (Fig. 8.3) further supports an association of calreticulin with the Ro/SS-A RNP.

Since the amino terminal amino acid sequence of this protein was unique and a synthetic peptide corresponding to this sequence was specifically reactive with anti-Ro/SS-A patient sera in ELISA,[12,18] we concluded that the 60-kDa polypeptide component of the Ro/SS-A RNP autoantigen had been identified (at that time the Ro/SS-A antigen was thought to consist of a single 60-kDa polypeptide that was bound to hYRNA molecules). A full-length cDNA encoding this anti-Ro/SS-A-reactive protein was subsequently isolated, cloned and sequenced in our lab by Daniel P. McCauliffe in collaboration with Marianna M. Newkirk, Ignacio Sanz, and J. Donald Capra.[19,20] The predicted amino acid sequence of this protein was found to share no significant homology with either the 52-kDa or 60-kDa Ro/SS-A proteins; however, it was extremely homologous to the sequences of rabbit and mouse calreticulin that had been reported at about that same time (data reviewed in ref. 21). Evidence was obtained in our lab which suggested that an affinity purified rabbit anti-calreticulin synthetic peptide antiserum could precipitate hYRNA, that native Wil-2 cell calreticulin was directly associated with RNA, and that a highly purified form of Wil-2 cell calreticulin reacted with the Center for Disease Control (CDC) anti-Ro/SS-A reference serum, AF/CDC7 by Western blot.[19] This information taken together ultimately led both ourselves[19,20] and others[22] to conclude that the human homologue of calreticulin had been isolated in our studies by virtue of its identity as a rheumatic disease-associated autoantigen (calreticulin had not previously been recognized to be associated with RNA or react with human autoantibody). In more recent studies, our lab has observed that only a subpopulation of Wil-2 cell calreticulin molecules appears to bind to hYRNA and reacts specifically with anti-Ro/SS-A sera.[23]

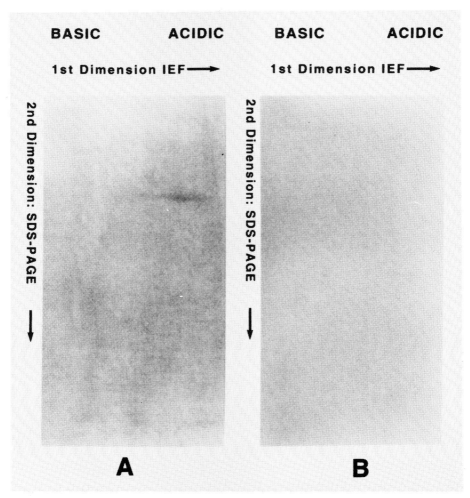

Fig. 8.2. Two dimensional immunoblot analysis of anti-Ro/SS-A autoantibody-reactive calreticulin fractions purified from Wil-2 cells. Samples resolved by 2D gels were electrophoretically transferred to nitrocellulose membrane in 25 mM Tris, 192 mM glycine buffer, 20% methanol, pH 8.3. The nitrocellulose was blocked with 1% bovine serum albumin in PBS-Tween for 1 h. The blots were then probed with (**A**) two rabbit anti-calreticulin synthetic peptide antisera (amino acids 7-28, 382-400) and (**B**) a rabbit anti-60-kDa Ro/SS-A synthetic peptide antiserum (amino acids 500-515) for 16 hours. The two rabbit anti-calreticulin synthetic peptide antisera were diluted 1:200 with 1% BSA in PBS-Tween while the anti-60-kDa Ro/SS-A synthetic peptide antiserum was similarly diluted 1:50. The blots were then washed with PBS-Tween 3 times and incubated with peroxidase conjugated goat anti-rabbit immunoglobulin (1:2000, TAGO) for 2 hours. The color was developed by reacting with diaminobenzidine tetrahydrochloride (12.5 mg/100 mg), 50 mM Tris, pH 7.6, and 1/10,000 volume of 30% H_2O_2. The color was developed by adding the substrate, 3,3'diaminobenzidine. The single band resulting from separation of the anti-Ro/SS-A-reactive Wil-2 cell calreticulin fraction in a 2D gel reacted with both anti-calreticulin synthetic peptide antisera (**A**) but not with the anti-60-kDa Ro/SS-A synthetic peptide antiserum (**B**).

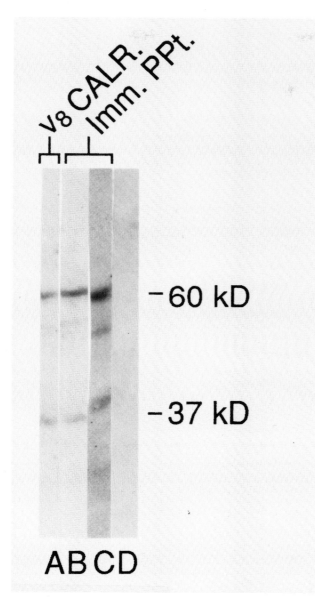

Fig. 8.3. $^{45}Ca^{2+}$ binding activity of a Ro/SS-A immunoprecipitate. An immunoprecipitate was produced by reacting a monospecific Ro/SS-A patient serum and polybuffer ion exchange column chromatography-derived fractions of Wil-2 cell extract in liquid phase immunoprecipitation at 4°C. The immunoprecipitate was then dissolved in SDS and treated with staphylococcal V-8 protease followed by analysis in a $^{45}Ca^{+2}$ overlay assay as described.[65] Briefly, the protease-digested immunoprecipitate was subjected to SDS-PAGE using 10% polyacrylamide at constant current for 70 min. The gels were electroblotted onto nitrocellulose membranes at constant current (0.5 amps) for 1.5 hours. The nitrocellulose membranes were initially washed at room temperatures for 2.5 hours in 5 mM imidazole pH 7.4 on a rotary shaker. The membranes were then incubated for 20 min in 20 ml of $^{45}Ca^{+2}$ overlay solution consisting of 5 mM imidazole, pH 7.4, 60 mM KCl, 5 mM $MgCl_2$, 10 µM nonradioactive Ca^{2+} and 1 µCi/ml $^{45}Ca^{2+}$ overlay solution. After incubation, the blots were thoroughly washed with 20 ml aliquots of chilled 30% absolute ethanol every 2 min for a total of 10 min, and then left to air dry completely. The membranes were exposed to Kodak X-OMAT AR film for 4 days at –70°C. Lane A: Staphylococcal V-8 protease digested purified Wil-2 cell calreticulin, lanes B and C: V-8 protease digested Ro/SS-A immunoprecipitates resulting from two 2 separate monospecific Ro/SS-A sera, lane D: immunoprecipitate resulting from a monospecific Sm patient serum. Both Ro/SS-A immunoprecipitates contained a Ca2+ binding protein that had a similar V-8 protease digestion pattern to calreticulin while the Sm immunoprecipitate did not.

In other studies, we cloned the human calreticulin gene and localized it to the short arm of chromosome 19.[19,20] The proximal calreticulin promoter sequence is similar enough to the promoters of the other endoplasmic reticulum luminal constituents (i.e., BiP [Grp78], endoplasmin [Grp94], protein disulfide isomerase) as to suggest that these genes might be co-regulated.[24] Endoplasmin (Grp94) has also been shown to be the target of autoantibody production in SLE patients.[25]

CONFIRMATION OF CALRETICULIN AS A NEW RHEUMATIC DISEASE AUTOANTIGEN

Several other laboratories have now confirmed that calreticulin is a new human rheumatic disease autoantigen. In 1991, Hunter et al[26] reported that an *E. coli*-produced recombinant form of human calreticulin reacted in ELISA with approximately 40% of the serum samples from unselected SLE patients. In that same year, Rokeach and coworkers[27] found that 33% of their SLE sera reacted with the an identical form of recombinant calreticulin by Western blot. In 1993, Kahlife et al[8] reported that SLE patients produce antibodies that react with the *Schistosoma mansoni* homologue of calreticulin in Western blots. In that same year, Conrad et al[28] found that a rat duodenal iron-binding homologue of calreticulin ("mobilferrin") reacted with anti-Ro/SS-A positive sera from SLE patients by dot-blot analysis. In addition, more recent studies by Boehm et al[25] have suggested that as many as 80% of SLE sera contain elevated levels of autoantibody that react with a purified form of native human liver calreticulin in ELISA. These same workers also found that SLE patients also produce autoantibody against another constituent of the endoplasmic reticulum, Grp94 (endoplasmin).

Other work has suggested that calreticulin autoantibodies can be found in a rather broad group of rheumatic diseases. In 1993, Routsias et al[29] confirmed earlier studies from our laboratory indicating that sera from patients with rheumatic disease frequently contain antibodies that react in ELISA to a synthetic peptide corresponding to the amino terminal of calreticulin.[12,18] This group reported that calreticulin amino-terminal peptide reactive antibodies could be found in 33% and 41% of their SLE and Sjögren's syndrome serum specimens respectively. Twenty-nine percent of their anti-Ro/SS-A and anti-Ro/SS-A:La/SS-B precipitating antibody-positive sera contained anti-calreticulin peptide antibodies.

Earlier studies in our lab had indicated that a higher percentage (~70%) of anti-Ro/SS-A precipitin-positive sera from subacute cutaneous LE and Sjögren's syndrome patients reacted in ELISA to a similar synthetic peptide.[18] The reason for the difference in these frequencies of reactivity is not altogether clear but could be technical (i.e., differences in the ELISA protocols) but more likely is related to differences in patient selection. Many of the anti-Ro/SS-A sera examined by Routsias et al[29] were from unselected SLE patients, whereas our LE patients were selected by virtue of having subacute cutaneous LE skin lesions. Routsias et al[29] also found calreticulin peptide reactive antibodies in disorders not commonly associated with the anti-Ro/SS-A autoantibody response (i.e., rheumatoid arthritis [25%], mixed connective tissue disease [28%]), supporting the possibility that antibodies reactive with calreticulin linear sequence epitopes might occur in a wider spectrum of rheumatic diseases, as has been suggested by others.[26,27] It remains to be determined whether different epitopes on calreticulin might be targeted in different rheumatic disease syndromes.

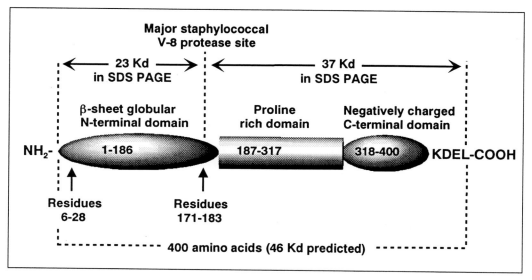

Fig. 8.4. *Summary of the present understanding of autoantibody binding sites on the calreticulin amino acid sequence. A diagramatic representation of the predicted secondary structure of the amino acid sequence of human calreticulin is shown as a three dimensional representation in the center of the figure. Treatment with staphlococcal V-8 protease under limiting digestion conditions cleaves this molecule into a 23-kDa N-terminal domain and a 37-kDa C-terminal domain as determined by SDS-PAGE. Autoantibodies present in LE and Sjögren's syndrome sera react predominately with the 23-kDa N-terminal domain by Western blot analysis. ELISA analysis using synthetic peptides corresponding to several portions of this sequence indicate that antibody binding sites reside in the regions of amino acid 6-28 and 171-183 (arrows at the bottom of the Figure). Amino acids 184-194 do not appear to contain an autoantibody binding site.*

QUESTIONS CONCERNING THE IDENTITY OF CALRETICULIN
AS A RO/SS-A AUTOANTIGEN

While it is now well established that calreticulin is a new human autoantigen, there has been considerable controversy over the past five years concerning the relationship that exists between calreticulin and the conventional components of the Ro/SS-A RNP. The ideas that calreticulin and Ro/SS-A autoantibody responses are positively correlated, that calreticulin can be precipitated by anti-Ro/SS-A sera in conjunction with other conventional components of the Ro/SS-A RNP, and that calreticulin is an hYRNA-binding protein have each been challenged.

Several groups have been unable to demonstrate a positive correlation between the presence of calreticulin autoantibody and conventional anti-Ro/SS-A autoantibody reactivity. While Hunter et al[26] and Rokeach et al[27] have identified calreticulin autoantibodies in SLE patient sera by ELISA and Western blot techniques respectively employing a prokaryotically-derived form of recombinant human calreticulin, this reactivity did not correlate positively with the presence of Ro/SS-A autoantibody activity in these same sera identified by conventional techniques.[26,27] In addition, Rokeach et al[27] could find none of 45 anti-Ro/SS-A sera they examined to react with *E. coli*-expressed recombinant calreticulin by Western blot. Also, this same group found that none of 35 anti-Ro/SS-A sera examined bound significantly to bacterially-expressed recombinant calreticulin in ELISA. In addition, none of 10 anti-Ro/SS-A sera including the CDC reference serum AF/CDC7 could be shown to react with bacterially-expressed recombinant calreticulin in Western blot by Pruijn et al.[30] Malhotra and co-workers[31] reported data suggesting that a native form of calreticulin purified from human spleen tissue reacted with anti-Ro/SS-A sera from Sjögren's syndrome patients by Western blot. However, this same group subsequently reported that this reactivity appeared to be directed toward the the 60-kDa component of the Ro/SS-A autoantigen that copurified with calreticulin.[32] While Boehm et al[25] found that a purified form of native human calreticulin reacted with 80% of their SLE sera by ELISA, they concluded that this reactivity was not associated with conventional anti-Ro/SS-A antibody activity.

In addition, several laboratories have been unable to immuno-precipitate various forms of calreticulin with anti-Ro/SS-A sera.

Rokeach et al[27] were unable to show that recombinant calreticulin translated in vitro in a rabbit reticulocyte system could be precipitated by 16 anti-Ro/SS-A patient sera or the anti-Ro/SS-A positive control serum (AF/CDC7) from the CDC. Pruijn et al[30] were unable to show that any of the 10 anti-Ro/SS-A sera examined reacted significantly with an in vitro translated form of calreticulin by immunoprecipitation. Boehm and coworkers[25] could not precipitate calreticulin from Hep-G2 cell extracts with several SLE sera that were capable of precipitating hYRNA from these same extracts.

Others have also been unable to identify a binding interaction between calreticulin and the Ro/SS-A RNP-associated hYRNAs. Rokeach et al[27] could not demonstrate that in vitro-translated calreticulin or *E. coli*-expressed recombinant calreticulin was associated with hY1RNA by immunoprecipitation or Northwestern blotting. In similar studies, Pruijn et al[30] were also unable to document an interaction between recombinant calreticulin and hYRNA. Boehm et al[25] were unable to demonstrate evidence of RNA associated with purified forms of rat, bovine, and human liver calreticulin. In addition, while SLE sera could be shown to immunoprecipitate hYRNA from radiolabeled Hep-G2 cell extracts, the same was not true for a rabbit antiserum raised against purified native human calreticulin.[25]

Possible Explanations for the Divergent Observations Concerning the Relationship Between Calreticulin and the Ro/SS-A RNP

We have observed that the cell line that has been used in virtually all of our studies (Wil-2) is a richer source of the autoantigenic form of calreticulin than other commonly used cell lines, such as Hela cells. It is possible that EB virus infection/transformation could potentiate the expression of the autoantigenic form of calreticulin. However, the autoantigenic form of calreticulin is not uniquely associated with EB virus infection since we have observed it in cell lines not infected with EB virus and in non-infected tissue such as normal human spleen, bovine brain, and guinea pig thyroid (personal observation).

We have observed that much of the autoantigenic activity of native calreticulin is quite labile under the denaturing conditions of standard Western blotting, which is often used by others to

identify the subcomponents of Ro/SS-A RNP particles (Table 8.1).
It is possible that the failure to identify calreticulin autoantibodies
in anti-Ro/SS-A sera by standard Western blot analysis by some
laboratories could relate to the fact that such autoantibodies are
directed in large part to conformational epitopes that are easily
disturbed by the denaturing conditions of the Western blot technique. In support of this possibility is the observation that conformational structure also appears to be critically important to the
autoantigenicity of the 60-kDa Ro/SS-A protein,[33] explaining the
poor reactivity of recombinant forms of 60-kDa Ro/SS-A protein
in Western blot.

Our more recent studies have indicated that only a subpopulation of cellular calreticulin molecules binds to hYRNA and interacts specifically with anti-Ro/SS-A sera.[23] Certain purification strategies might be more efficient than others in separating this fraction
of calreticulin molecules from the relatively large total cellular pool
of calreticulin. It is also possible that calreticulin molecules are
not associated with all Ro/SS-A RNP particles or that they associated with such particles only transiently, as do La/SS-B molecules.

Some workers have argued that copurification of calreticulin
with the 60-kDa Ro/SS-A protein could account for an "apparent" association between calreticulin and the Ro/SS-A RNP
autoantigen.[32] It is well known that the amino terminal of purified native forms of 60-kDa Ro/SS-A protein is blocked, preventing conventional sequencing of this protein. Thus, sequencing of
a mixture of 60-kDa Ro/SS-A and calreticulin would yield only
the amino acid sequence of calreticulin. While it is certainly true
that calreticulin purified by some protocols might be contaminated
by the 60-kDa Ro/SS-A protein, native Wil-2 cell calreticulin purified by the protocol that has been employed in our laboratory is
not so contaminated (Fig. 8.1 and 8.2). Therefore, we do not feel
that such an explanation for the association that we have observed
between calreticulin and the Ro/SS-A RNP is valid.

We, like others, have had difficulty demonstrating specific reactivity of anti-Ro/SS-A sera with unmodified forms of E. *coli*-
and baculovirus-produced recombinant human calreticulin. As is
true of the conventional Ro/SS-A RNP,[33] much of the autoantibody reactivity of native calreticulin derived from Wil-2 cells is
dependent on conformational structure and is easily lost in denaturing assays such as a standard Western blot. Thus, it is not

surprising that unmodified forms of prokaryotic recombinant calreticulin fail to react optimally with calreticulin autoantibody present in Ro/SS-A sera. Our current working hypothesis is that some form of post-translational modification, possibly involving phosphorylation, is required to provide the fully autoantigenic configuration of calreticulin. It is possible that conformation shifts in calreticulin secondary to its association with hYRNA are also important to the autoantigenicity of this molecule.

Recently published studies by others have now firmly documented that calreticulin is capable of binding to RNA even in the absence of an RNP concensus sequence. Hira L. Nakhasi and coworkers[34-37] (Chapter 7) have demonstrated that phosphorylated calreticulin binds specifically to a 3'(+) stem-loop structure on rubella genomic RNA that is involved in the replication of rubella virus within mammalian cells. Moreover, recent experiments in our lab have demonstrated that calreticulin unequivocally and specifically binds to all four species of hYRNA in gel mobility shift assay by a mechanism that does not appear to be as fully dependent on phosphorylation as does the binding of rubella RNA.[38] It is somewhat difficult to understand why the earlier studies by Rokeach et al[27] did not demonstrate hY1RNA binding to calreticulin since the same hY1RNA plasmid was used in both sets of studies. It is possible that the assays used by these workers (immunoprecipitation and Northwestern blotting) were less sensitive than the electrophoretic gel mobility shift assay used in our studies. Furthermore, the recombinant calreticulin constructs used in these two studies also differed somewhat.

EPITOPE MAPPING OF CALRETICULIN

Studies have begun to address which specific regions of the calreticulin amino acid sequence are targeted by the autoimmune response against this molecule that is seen in rheumatic disease sera. Preliminary antibody inhibition studies employing a rabbit antiserum raised against a synthetic peptide corresponding to the amino acids 6-19 of this molecule indicated that the N-terminal region of calreticulin contained a major autoepitope.[12] Protease digestion mapping studies have also supported this idea. When native Wil-2 cell calreticulin is treated with staphylococcal V-8 protease under limiting conditions, the molecule can be cleaved into a 23-kDa N-terminal domain and a 37-kDa C-terminal domain as determined by SDS-PAGE.[18] Our group has found that much of the autoantibody activity contained in anti-Ro/SS-A antibody-positive rheumatic disease sera is directed toward the N-terminal 23-kDa domain of this molecule.[14] Calreticulin autoantibodies present in onchocerciasis sera appear to react with this molecule in a more complex manner.[14]

The importance of the N-terminal region of this molecule to its autoantibody-binding activity has been further supported by ELISA studies employing synthetic peptides corresponding to this region. Computer algorithm analysis predicted that an antibody binding site was likely contained within the first 30 amino acids of the fully processed form of this molecule.[19] The initial studies with a synthetic peptide corresponding to amino acids 6-19 of human calreticulin indicated that autoantibodies present in anti-Ro/SS-A sera reacted specifically with this sequence in ELISA.[12] Similar results were found with a related synthetic peptide corresponding to amino acids 7-24.[18] This latter study also indicated that some other regions of the human calreticulin amino acid sequence (e.g., 171-183) also react with anti-Ro/SS-A sera whereas others (e.g., 184-194) do not.[18] As discussed above, while other workers have documented that rheumatic disease sera frequently contain autoantibody activity directed toward calreticulin N-terminal synthetic peptides, this autoantibody activity has not been confirmed to be specifically related to the anti-Ro/SS-A autoantibody response.[29]

Whether different epitopes on calreticulin are targeted in different autoimmune disease states in which autoantibody production to this molecule occurs remains to be confirmed. However, preliminary ELISA studies employing several synthetic peptides have suggested that this might be the case.[18]

ROLE PLAYED BY THE CALRETICULIN AUTOIMMUNE RESPONSE IN RO/SS-A AUTOANTIBODY-ASSOCIATED CUTANEOUS LE

A fundamental hypothesis being tested in our laboratory is that autoantibodies present in Ro/SS-A autoimmune sera participate in the pathogenesis of the characteristic pattern of epidermal cell injury that is seen in photosensitive LE-specific skin lesions such as subacute cutaneous LE and neonatal LE.[39,40] Since previous studies in our lab have indicated that autoantibodies to native forms of calreticulin are produced in parallel to the classical anti-Ro/SS-A autoimmune response, we have become quite interested in the prospect that an autoimmune response to calreticulin might be involved in the pathogenesis of anti-Ro/SS-A autoantibody-associated forms of cutaneous LE such as subacute cutaneous LE and neonatal LE.

Ultraviolet light (UVB)-induced cell surface expression of Ro/SS-A autoantigens in epidermal keratinocytes has been implicated in the pathogenesis of photosensitive, Ro/SS-A autoantibody-associated skin lesions such as subacute cutaneous LE and neonatal LE.[41-44] One group has suggested that this pattern of cell surface Ro/SS-A autoantigen expression might occur as the result of UVB-induced apoptosis.[45] Exposure to UVB radiation also appears to be capable of inducing the expression of calreticulin on the plasma membrane of lymphoblastoid cells[48] epidermal keratinocyte lines,[2,3] and normal human keratinocytes.[47] Work has also suggested that calreticulin expression at the cell surface of epidermal keratinocytes following UVB irradiation might occur as the result of UVB-induced apoptosis.[48] Studies in our own lab have also suggested that UVB irradiation can also increase cellular calreticulin antigen levels and mRNA levels in transformed human epidermal keratinocytes.[2] As with the conventional components of Ro/SS-A autoantigen, expression of the autoantigenic form of calreticulin on the plasma membrane could target cells such as epidermal keratinocytes for immune-mediated injury in those individuals who produce autoantibodies or specific T cell responses against this molecule. Cellular infection with the cytomegalovirus has also been reported to induce cell surface expression of calreticulin.[49]

CALRETICULIN AUTOIMMUNITY IN HUMAN PARASITIC DISEASE

The filarial homologues of calreticulin appear to be immunodominant antigens targeted by protective immune responses generated in humans suffering from onchocerciasis[6,7] and shistosomiasis.[8,50] The high degree of sequence homology between human calreticulin and the *O. volvulvs*[51] and *S. mansoni*[8] forms of calreticulin, combined with the observation that calreticulin is a human autoantigen, has led to the suggestion that a component of the tissue injury that occurs in diseases such as onchocerciasis and shistosomiasis might result from a cross reactive autoimmune response to calreticulin.[52,53] In support of this hypothesis are the observations that patients with onchocerciasis have been shown to produce antibodies that crossreact with native and recombinant human calreticulin[27,52,54] and that serum from patients with SLE contains antibody that reacts with the *S. mansoni* form of calreticulin.[8]

CALRETICULIN AUTOIMMUNITY IN AUTOIMMUNE LIVER DISEASE

Antibodies against a drug-altered form of calreticulin are produced in halothane hepatitis and animal models of spontaneous autoimmune hepatitis.[55] The role played by such autoantibodies in the pathogenesis of autoimmune hepatocyte injury has not yet been determined.

POTENTIAL MECHANISMS BY WHICH CALRETICULIN MIGHT BE TARGETED BY THE AUTOIMMUNE RESPONSE

As with most rheumatic disease autoantigens, the reason(s) why calreticulin is targeted by an autoimmune response is not at all clear. However, there is increasing evidence to suggest that molecular mimicry is one mechanism by which such autoimmune responses might be explained (data reviewed in ref. 56). The fundamental idea is that crossreactive immune responses against self molecules are generated as the result of a genetically-determined dysregulated immune response against highly homologous molecules encoded by human pathogens, especially viruses. There is increasing evidence to suggest that a microbe-generated crossreactive immune response against a single component of a linked set of polypeptides and RNA molecules such as the hYRNA RNP could eventually lead to autoantibody responses to multiple components of such particles through mechanisms of epitope spreading and affinity maturation.[57] There is much suspicion that such crossreactive autoantibody responses are orchestrated by autoantigen-specific T cells, although the existence of such cells has often been very difficult to prove.

Recent work has suggested that certain viruses interact with mammalian host cell calreticulin molecules in a way that could serve to target them for autoimmune attack. Rubella virus infection increases cellular levels of phosphorylated calreticulin.[34,35] This form of calreticulin appears to be a critical host response protein that interacts with a controlling element of rubella genomic RNA that is essential for rubella virus replication.[37,58] Hira Nakhasi and colleagues[36,58] in an elegant series of studies have shown that a phosphorylated, E. coli-expressed recombinant human calreticulin fusion protein binds to a 3' stem-loop structure of rubella genomic RNA. This protein-RNA binding interaction appears to be completely dependent upon phosphorylation. Thus, a post-translationally modified form of calreticulin, by interacting with a critical regulatory element within the rubella genome, appears to be involved in intracellular replication of some types of RNA viruses. A related virus, sindbis, appears to interact with calreticulin in a similar manner during its replication cycle.[35] Using electrophoretic mobility shift analysis, our lab has recently found that a human calreticulin fusion protein produced in E.coli binds specifically to all four species of hYRNA in the apparent absence of exogenous phosphorylation, suggesting a different binding mechanism than that used by rubella genomic RNA.[38] The recent observations that another conventional component of the Ro/SS-A RNP, the La/SS-B protein, functionally interacts with regulatory RNA stem-loop structures present in polio[59,60] and HIV-1[61,62] viruses is of additional interest in this regard.

Hira Nakhasi's group[63] has also reported that anti-Ro/SS-A sera precipitate 60- and 52-kDa proteins (the identities of which have yet to be fully confirmed) that bind to a stem-loop structure present on the 5'(+) end of rubella genomic RNA that is involved in the control of translation of rubella proteins. This observation suggests that other components of the Ro/SS-A RNP particle might be involved in the replication of rubella virus within mammalian cells. Also of note in this regard is the observation that infection with a closely related RNA virus, sindbis, induces the expression of Ro/SS-A antigens and fragments of the endoplasmic reticulum, including calreticulin, in association with viral antigens in surface blebs of cells undergoing apoptosis.[48]

There is currently little evidence that an autoimmune response to calreticulin is generated during the course of infection with rubella or sindbis viruses, although systematic studies in this area have not yet been reported. In preliminary collaborative studies with Dr. Paul E. Phillips at the SUNY Health Science Center, our lab has identified precipitating antibody to purified Wil-2 cell calreticulin by CIE in 3/6 serum specimens from individuals whose rubella serology became positive following immunization with the RA 27/3 vaccine (unpublished observation). However, much additional work is needed to determine the true role played by viral infection in the generation of calreticulin autoimmunity.

It is also possible that a crossreactive immune response to the highly homologous forms of calreticulin that are expressed by higher forms of human pathogens such as *O. volvulus* and *S. mansoni* could be involved in the generation of calreticulin autoantibodies that are found in the human diseases caused by these organisms.

SUMMARY

Among the many intriguing biological facets of the calreticulin amino acid sequence is that of a human autoantigen. While debate continues concerning the relationship that calreticulin shares with the Ro/SS-A autoantigen, there is now little doubt that calreticulin is frequently targeted by autoantibody production in a number of the rheumatic diseases including SLE and several of its subsets (subacute cutaneous LE, neonatal LE), Sjögren's syndrome, rheumatoid arthritis, and mixed connective tissue disease. The role that autoimmune responses to calreticulin might play in the pathogenesis of such disorders remains to be explored. In addition, autoantibody responses to calreticulin have been documented in human parasitic disease including onchocerciasis and shistosomiasis as well as autoimmune forms of hepatitis. The mechanisms responsible for autoimmune responses to calreticulin have for the most part not been explored. However, as with many other human rheumatic disease autoantigens, the concept that dysregulated crossreactive immune responses to highly-conserved microbial antigens (i.e., molecular mimicry) is receiving increasing attention as a mechanism that might explain such patterns of autoimmune response. Recent observations demonstrating an interaction between post-translationally modified forms of calreticulin and rubella/sindbis viruses have fueled speculation that some forms of the calreticulin autoimmune response could also be the result of molecular mimicry.

ACKNOWLEDGMENTS

This work was supported by NIH grants AR19101, AI12127, and the resources of the U.T. Southwestern Skin Disease Research Core Center (AR41940). We wish to thank Dr. Frank Arnett

(University of Texas Health Science Center at Houston), Dr. Lela Lee (University of Oklahoma Health Sciences Center), Dr. David Norris (University of Colorado Health Sciences Center), and Dr. Jay-Shong Deng (University of Pittsburgh School of Medicine) for generously sharing their anti-Ro/SS-A patient sera with us.

REFERENCES

1. Sontheimer RD, Lieu T-S, Capra JD. The diverse functional repertoire of calreticulin, a new human autoantigen. The Immunologist 1993; 1:155-160.
2. Kawashima T, Lieu T-S, Zappi E et al. Regulation of expression of the polypeptide constituents of the Ro autoantigen complex in transformed human epidermal keratinocytes. Lupus 1994; 3:493-500.
3. Kawashima T, Zappi EG, Lieu T-S et al. Impact of ultraviolet radiation on the cellular expression of Ro/SS-A-autoantigenic polypeptides. Dermatology 1994; 189:6-10.
4. Gersten DM, Bijwaard KE, Law LW et al. Homology of the B50 melanoma antigen to the Ro/SS-A antigen of human systemic LE and calcium binding proteins. Biochim Biophys Acta 1991; 1096:20-25.
5. Bijwaard K, Vieira WD, Leiu TS et al. Studies on the expression and immunogenicity of the B50 melanoma antigen and its relationship to calreticulin. Melanoma Res 1995; (in press).
6. Unnasch TR, Gallin MY, Soboslay PT et al. Isolation and characterization of expression cDNA clones encoding antigens of *Onchocerca volvulus* infective larvae. J Clin Invest 1988; 82:262-269.
7. Lux FA, McCauliffe DP, Buttner DW et al. Serological cross-activity between a human Ro autoantigen (calreticulin) and the lambda Ral-1 antigen of *Onchocerca volvulas*. J Clin Invest 1992; 89:1945-1951.
8. Khalife J, Trottein F, Schacht A-M et al. Cloning of the gene encoding a *Schistosoma mansoni* antigen homologous to human Ro/SS-A autoantigen. Mol Biochem Parasitol 1993; 57:193-202.
9. Zappi E, Sontheimer R. Clinical relevance of antibodies to Ro/SS-A and La/SS-B in subacute cutaneous lupus erythematosus and related conditions. Immunol Invest 1993; 22:189-203.
10. McCauliffe DP, Sontheimer RD. Molecular characterization of the Ro/SS-A autoantigens. J Invest Dermatol 1993; 100: 73S-79S.
11. Lieu T-S, Jiang M, Steigerwald JC et al. Identification of the SS-A/Ro intracellular antigen with autoimmune sera. J Immunol Methods 1984; 71:217-228.
12. Lieu T-S, Newkirk M, Capra JD et al. Molecular characterization of human Ro/SS-A antigen: amino terminal sequence of the protein moiety of human Ro/SS-A antigen and immunological activity to a corresponding synthetic peptide. J Clin Invest 1988; 82:96-101.

13. Lieu T-S, McCauliffe DP, Newkirk MM et al. A major autoepitope is present on the amino terminus of the human Ro/SS-A polypeptide. J Autoimmunity 1989; 2:367-374.

14. Lux FA, McCauliffe DP, Buttner DW et al. Serological cross-reactivity between a human Ro/SS-A autoantigen (calreticulin) and the lambda Ral-1 antigen of *Onchocerca volvulus*. J Clin Invest 1992; 89:1945-1951.

15. Deutscher SL, Harley JB, Keene JD. Molecular analysis of the 60 kD human Ro ribonucleoprotein. Proc Natl Acad Sci USA 1988; 85:9479-9483.

16. Chan EKL, Hamel JC, Peebles CL et al. Molecular characterization and cloning of the 52 kDa SS-A/Ro protein. Mol Biol Rep 1990; 14:53-53.

17. Itoh K, Itoh Y, Frank MB. Protein heterogeneity in the human Ro/SSA ribonucleoproteins. The 52- and 60-kD Ro/SSA autoantigens are encoded by separate genes. J Clin Invest 1991; 87:177-186.

18. Lieu TS, Newkirk MM, Arnett FC et al. A major autoepitope is present on the amino terminus of a human SS-A/Ro polypeptide. J Autoimmunity 1989; 2:367-374.

19. McCauliffe DP, Lux FA, Lieu T-S et al. Molecular cloning, expression, and chromosome 19 localization of a human Ro/SS-A autoantigen. J Clin Invest 1990; 85:1379-1391.

20. McCauliffe DP, Zappi E, Lieu T-S et al. A human Ro/SS-A autoantigen is the homologue of calreticulin and is highly homologous with onchocercal RAL-1 antigen and an aplysia "memory molecule". J Clin Invest 1990; 86:332-335.

21. Michalak M, Milner RE, Burns K et al. Calreticulin. Biochem J 1992; 285:681-692.

22. Collins JH, Xi ZJ, Alderson-Lang BH et al. Sequence homology of a canine brain calcium-binding protein with calregulin and the human Ro/SS-A antigen. Biochem Biophys Res Commun 1989; 164:575-579.

23. Lieu TS, Sontheimer RD. A subpopulation of Wil-2 cell calreticulin molecules is found within Ro/SS-A ribonucleoprotein particles. Submitted for publication, 1995.

24. McCauliffe DP, Yang YS, Wilson J et al. The 5'-flanking region of the human calreticulin gene shares homology with the human GRP78, GRP94, and protein disulfide isomerase promoters. J Biol Chem 1992; 267: 2557-2562.

25. Boehm J, Orth T, Van Nguyen P et al. Systemic lupus erythematosus is associated with increased auto-antibody titers against calreticulin and Grp94, but calreticulin is not the Ro/SS-A antigen. Eur J Clin Invest 1994; 24:248-257.

26. Hunter FA, Barger BD, Schrohenloher R et al. Autoantibodies to carlreticulin in the sera of systemic lupus erythematosus. Arthritis Rheum 1991; 34: S75.

27. Rokeach LA, Haselby JA, Meilof JF et al. Characterization of the autoantigen calreticulin. J Immunol 1991; 147:3031-3039.
28. Conrad ME, Umbreit JN, Moore EG. Rat duodenal iron-binding protein mobiferrin is a homologue of calreticulin. Gastroenterology 1993; 104:1700-1704.
29. Routsias JG, Tzioufas AG, Sakarellos-Daitsiotis M et al. Calreticulin synthetic peptide analogues: anti-peptide antibodies in autoimmune rheumatic diseases. Clin Exp Immunol 1993; 91:437-441.
30. Pruijn GJ, Bozic B, Schoute F et al. Redefined definition of the 56K and other autoantigens in the 50-60 KDa region. Mol Biol Rep 1992; 16:267-276.
31. Malhotra R, Willis AC, Jensenius JC et al. Structure and homology of the human C1q receptor (collectin receptor). Immunology 1993; 78:341-348.
32. Lu J, Willis AC, Sim RB. A calreticulin-like protein co-purifies with a '60 kD' component of Ro/SSA, but is not recognized by antibodies in Sjogren's syndrome sera. Clin Exp Immunol 1993; 94:429-434.
33. Itoh Y, Reichlin M. Autoantibodies to the Ro/SS-A antigen confirmation dependent. 1: Anti-60-kD antibodies are mainly directed to the native protein; anti-52 kD antibodies are mainly directed to the denatured protein. Autoimmunity 1992; 14:57-65.
34. Nakhasi HL, Rouault TA, Haile DJ, et al. Specific high affinity binding of host cell proteins to the 3' region of rubella virus RNA. New Biologist 1990; 2:255-264.
35. Nakhasi HL, Cao XQ, Rouault TA et al. Specific binding of host cell proteins to the 3'-terminal serum loop structure to rubella virus negative-strand RNA. J Virol 1991; 65:5961-5967.
36. Nakhasi HL, Singh NK, Pogue GP et al. Identification and characterization of host factor interactions with cis-acting elements of rubella virus RNA. Arch Virol 1994; 9:255-267.
37. Singh NK, Atreya CD, Nakhasi HL. Identification of calreticulin as a rubella virus RNA binding protein. Proc Natl Acad Sci USA 1994; 91:12770-12774.
38. Cheng ST, Nguyen TQ, Capra JD et al. Recombinant calreticulin binds specifically to synthetic hYRNA (abstract). J Invest Dermatol 1995; 104:653.
39. Sontheimer RD, McCauliffe DP. Pathogenesis of anti-Ro/SS-A autoantibody-associated cutaneous lupus erythematosus. Dermatol Clin 1990; 8:751-758.
40. Norris DA. Pathomechanisms of photosensitive lupus erythematosus. J Invest Dermatol 1993; 100:58S-68S.
41. LeFeber WP, Norris DA, Ryan SR et al. Ultraviolet light induces binding of antibodies to selected nuclear antigens on cultured human keratinocytes. J Clin Invest 1984; 74:1545-1551.

42. Furukawa F, Kashihara-Sawami M, Lyons MB et al. Binding of antibodies to the extractable nuclear antigens SS-A/Ro and SS-B/La is induced on the surface of human keratinocytes by ultraviolet light (UVL): Implications for the pathogenesis of photosensitive cutaneous lupus. J Invest Dermatol 1990; 94:77-85.

43. Jones SK. Ultraviolet radiation (UVR) induces cell-surface Ro/SSA antigen expression by human keratinocytes in vitro: A possible mechanism for the UVR induction of cutaneous lupus lesions. Br J Dermatol 1992; 126:546-553.

44. Golan TD, Elkon KB, Gharavi AE et al. Enhanced membrane binding of autoantigens to cultured keratinocytes of systemic lupus erythematosus patients after ultraviolet B/ultraviolet A irradiation. J Clin Invest 1992; 90:1067.

45. Casciola-Rosen LA, Anhalt G, Rosen A. Autoantigens targeted in systemic lupus erythematosus are clustered in two populations of surface structures on apoptotic keratinocytes. J Exp Med 1994; 179:1317-1330.

46. Newkirk MM, Tsoukas C. Effect of ultraviolet irradiation on selected host cell proteins including Ro/SS-A and Epstein-Barr virus in cultured lymphoblastoid cell lines. J Autoimmunity 1992; 5:511-525.

47. Zhu J. Cytomegalovirus infection induces expression of 60 kD/Ro antigen on human keratinocytes. Lupus 1995; (in press)

48. Rosen A, Casciola-Rosen L, Ahearn J. Novel packages of viral and self antigens are generated during apoptosis. J Exp Med 1995; 181:1557-1561.

49. Zhu J, Newkirk MM. Viral induction of the human autoantigen calreticulin. Clin Invest Med 1994; 17:196-205.

50. Hawn TR, Tom TD, Strand M. Molecular cloning and expression of SmIrV1, a *Schistosoma mansoni* antigen with similarity to calnexin, calreticulin, and OvRal1. J Biol Chem 1993; 268:7692-7698.

51. McCauliffe DP, Zappi E, Lieu TS et al. A human Ro/SS-A autoantigen is the homologue of calreticulin and is highly homologous with onchocercal RAL-1 antigen and an aplysia "memory molecule". J Clin Invest 1990; 86:332-335.

52. Lux FA, McCauliffe DP, Büttner DW et al. Serological cross-reactivity between a human Ro/SS-A autoantigen (calreticulin) and the lambdaRAL-1 antigen of *Onchocerca volvulus*. J Clin Invest 1992; 89:1945-1951.

53. Zhou Y, Dziak E, Unnasch TR et al. Major retinal cell components recognized by onchocerciasis sera are associated with the cell surface and nucleoli. Invest Ophthal Vis Sci 1994; 35:1089-1099.

54. Meilof JF, Van der Lelij A, Rokeach LA et al. Autoimmunity and filariasis. Autoantibodies against cytoplasmic cellular proteins in sera of patients with onchocerciasis. J Immunol 1993; 151:5800-5809.

55. Yokoi T, Nagayama S, Kajiwara R et al. Identification of protein disulfide isomerase and calreticulin as autoimmune antigens in LEC strain of rats. Biochim Biophys Acta 1993; 1158:339-344.

56. Behar SM, Porcelli SA. Mechanisms of autoimmune disease induction. The role of the immune response to microbial pathogens. Arthritis Rheum 1995; 38:458-476.

57. Huang S-C, Pan Z, Kurien BT et al. Immunization with vesicular stomatitis virus nucleocapsid protein induces autoantibodies to the 60 KD Ro/SS-A ribonucleoprotein particle. J Invest Med 1995; 43:151-158.

58. Nakhasi HL, Singh NK, Pogue GP et al. Identification and characterization of host factor interactions with cis-acting elements of rubella virus RNA. Arch Virol 1994; 9:255-267.

59. Meerovitch K, Svitkin YV, Lee HS et al. La autoantigen enhances and corrects aberrant translation of polio virus RNA in reticulocytic lysate. J Virol 1993; 67:3798-3807.

60. Svitkin YV, Meerovitch K, Lee HS et al. Internal translation initiation on poliovirus RNA: Further characterization of La function in poliovirus translation in vitro. J Virol 1994; 68:1544-1550.

61. Svitkin YV, Pause A, Sonenberg N. La autoantigen alleviates translational repression by the 5' leader sequence of the human immunodeficiency virus type 1 mRNA. J Virol 1994; 68:7001-7007.

62. Chang Y-N, Kenan DJ, Keene JD et al. Direct interactions between autoantigen La and human immunodeficiency virus leader RNA. J Virol 1994; 68:7008-7020.

63. Pogue GP, Cao XQ, Singh NK et al. 5' sequences of rubella virus RNA stimulate translation of chimeric RNA's and specifically interact with two host encoded proteins. J Virol 1993; 67:7106-7117.

64. Tobwin HT, Staehelin T, Gordon J. Electrophoretic transfer of proteins from polyacrylamide gels to nitrocellulose sheets: procedure and some applications. Proc Natl Acad Sci USA 1979; 76:4350.

65. Maruyama K, Mikawa T, Ebashi S. Detection of calcium binding proteins by ^{45}Ca autoradiography on nitrocellulose membrane after sodium dodecyl sulfate gel electrophoresis. J Biochem (Tokyo) 1984; 95:511-519.

CHAPTER 9

CALRETICULIN IN T LYMPHOCYTES

R. Chris Bleackley, Michael J. Pinkoski and Eric A. Atkinson

INTRODUCTION

Calreticulin was originally described as a Ca^{2+} binding protein found in the sarcoplasmic reticulum.[1] Since its discovery the majority of experiments have focused on a potential role in regulating Ca^{2+} levels within this organelle. Why then should the protein turn up in the nucleus,[2] or associated with integrins,[3] or even in the blood stream of individuals with river blindness?[4] Could the protein play a variety of roles in different cell types that has been ignored because of the bias implied by the initial description? Our own thinking on this subject was influenced by our discovery that the steady state levels of calreticulin mRNA and protein were drastically upregulated after T lymphocyte stimulation.[5] Why should an activated immune cell need to upregulate a Ca^{2+} binding protein? The majority of readers have likely forgotten more immunology than they care to acknowledge, so before we can address this question a short review of some of the essential features of the immune system will be presented.

OVERVIEW OF THE IMMUNE SYSTEM

There are two branches to the immune system. Humoral immunity is mediated by B lymphocytes that produce antibodies after stimulation by foreign molecules (antigens). These antibodies then bind to the antigenic structures and neutralize them or enhance their recognition, uptake and ultimate destruction by phagocytic cells such as macrophages. This arm of the immune system serves to protect us against bacteria and toxins. The effectors of cell mediated immunity are the T lymphocytes. They defend us against virus infected and tumor cells, and are involved in rejection of grafted organs. Like B cells, T lymphocytes have the ability to recognize and respond to antigenic or foreign structures. In the case of T cells this is achieved via the T cell antigen receptor (TCR), while B cells utilize a membrane form of immunoglobulin to bind the foreign structures. However, in the case of T lymphocytes the antigen must be "presented" on the surface of a cell. For the initiation of a response, antigens are broken down into peptides and presented on the surface of a specialist antigen-presenting cell (APC; e.g. macrophage). Once the T cells have been activated they can recognize the foreign molecules on the surface of the virus infected or tumor cell and thus engineer the demise of this potentially harmful cell. Foreign molecules are not recognized in isolation but are seen by the T cell antigen receptor in the context of major histocompatibility antigens. Consequently, most T cell responses are specific to both the antigen and the MHC type (this is known as MHC restriction). During their maturation in the thymus, the developing T cells are selected for on the basis of their ability to recognize self MHC and inability to respond to self-antigens. After attending school in the thymus they emerge as educated cells that are now able to respond to antigen-MHC structures and become functional T lymphocytes.

T CELL SUBSETS

A variety of different subsets of T lymphocytes have now been characterized. For the sake of simplicity we will restrict our discussion to helper (TH) and cytotoxic cells (CTL). The majority of helper cells respond to antigens in the context of class II MHC because they have on their surface a protein named CD4 that can bind to this class of MHC. In contrast, many cytotoxic T cells express CD8 rather than CD4, and thus bind to class I MHC-antigen complexes. As a general rule these TH cells respond to antigen presented on the surface of MHC class II positive APCs, by transcribing, translating and secreting a variety of soluble growth/differentiation/migratory factors known as lymphokines. Cytotoxic T lymphocytes bind to antigen–class I MHC and as a consequence of new gene expression become responsive to some of the lymphokines produced by the TH. After binding of the lymphokine to the high affinity receptor on the surface, the CTL is driven through the final steps of activation. New genes are expressed in the CTL that encode the molecules which will ultimately be responsible for the ability of this activated cell to destroy its target. In addition these cells proliferate and are released into the circulation to allow them to seek out and destroy the invaders. This simplified view of T cell activation will serve as a useful framework for the discussions in this chapter. The reader should realize, however, that real life is not so black and white. Some helper cells can kill and lymphokines can be produced by CTL.[6,7] In addition other "costimulatory"[8] and adherence molecules play major roles in T lymphocyte activation.[9]

T LYMPHOCYTE ACTIVATION

When a T lymphocyte is activated upon engagement of its antigen receptor a series of events occur that result in the transmission of the signal from the cytoplasmic membrane through the cytoplasm into the nucleus with resultant induction of specific gene expression. Early stages of this transduction involve activation and clustering of tyrosine kinases, hydrolysis of phosphoinositides and an increase in intracellular Ca^{2+} (100 nM to 1 μM). The elevated free Ca^{2+} is bound by a number of Ca^{2+} binding effector proteins that are essential for subsequent phosphorylation cascades involving specific transcription factors and cytoskeletal reorganization. Thus control of free cytoplasmic Ca^{2+} levels is of paramount importance in mediating T cell activation. The increase appears to have two components, an early peak that lasts for around 2 minutes and then a plateau that can be maintained for an hour.[10,11] The early peak is not affected by chelation of extracellular Ca^{2+} whereas the late phase is.[12,13] It is believed that Ca^{2+} is initially released from intracellular organelles via the InsP$_3$ receptor which acts as a Ca^{2+} release channel. The later plateau is achieved by extracellular influx. Similar results have been seen with bulk and individual cells, although in the recordings taken from single cells oscillations rather than peaks are observed. The basis of these oscillations is not understood but is discussed elsewhere.[14,15] Obviously Ca^{2+} binding proteins are extremely important in this process. The specific role of calreticulin has not been examined but its presence within the endoplasmic reticulum, a likely although not proven target for the InsP$_3$ receptor channel, implicates it as a potential source of Ca^{2+} for the early flux. Recent results have suggested that T lymphocyte activation is also associated with Ca^{2+} stores outside, as well as within, the endoplasmic reticulum.[16]

This suggests a role for the calreticulin that is present in T lymphocytes prior to activation, but what of the dramatic increase in calreticulin mRNA and protein seen after TCR engagement? We would submit that this newly synthesized protein is fulfilling a completely different function in the activated T cell. Certainly the kinetics would argue against a role for new calreticulin in the activation process itself; with a signal needing to be transduced to activate the calreticulin gene before any protein can be produced! Secondly, as CTL are stimulated calreticulin appears primarily in the cytoplasmic granules;[17] the organelle that has been implicated as carrying the effector molecules of CTL-mediated target cell destruction.

CTL-MEDIATED LYSIS OF TARGET CELLS

Once the CTL has been activated it can then bind to and destroy any cell that expresses the stimulating antigen in the context of the correct class I MHC. The mechanism(s) by which lysis of the target cell is achieved has been the subject of intensive research over the last few years. From the point of view of the target it appears that the primary mechanism to explain its demise is the induction of the apoptotic or programmed cell death pathway by the CTL. Morphologically the target cells do appear to be undergoing apoptosis and the biochemical hallmark of this process, DNA fragmentation, is often observed.[18] In contrast to many descriptions of apoptosis, during development or in response to hormones for example, CTL-induced death does not require protein synthesis or transcription of new genes within the target cell prior to cell death.

The means by which the CTL induces apoptosis is somewhat controversial and a number of mechanisms have been suggested.[19] These include the production of cytolytic factors by the CTL,[20,21] the granule-mediated mechanism and the Fas-antigen mediated pathway.[22,23] Here we will describe the granule-mediated mechanism, as the present evidence would suggest that this is where calreticulin may play an important role. It should be realized, however, that Ca^{2+} has been implicated in other mechanisms and thus, *vide infra,* a Ca^{2+} binding protein such as calreticulin may be implicated.

Activated cytotoxic T lymphocytes contain cytoplasmic granules. Shortly after making contact with the target cell, through specific interactions between the TCR and antigen/MHC, a wave of Ca^{2+} fluxes is seen and there is a reorganization within the cytoplasm of the CTL.[24] The microtubule organizing centre and the Golgi apparatus reorient toward, and the granules appear to move toward, the point of contact with the target cell.[25] Thus, this vectoral exocytosis is believed to deliver the lytic effector molecules at high concentration in the vicinity of the target cell.[26] Ever since it was discovered that the granules themselves are able to induce lysis in cells, these organelles have become the focus of the search for cytolytic effector molecules.[27-29] Granules can be obtained from killer cells by nitrogen cavitation and Percoll gradient fractionation. As with whole cells, granule-mediated lysis is rapid and is accompanied by DNA fragmentation in the target cell. Both lysis and fragmentation are dependent on the presence of Ca^{2+} at the time of lysis although preincubation of granules with Ca^{2+}, prior to their addition to targets, abrogates lytic activity.[29]

MOLECULES IN CTL GRANULES

A number of molecules have been isolated from granules, including perforin, granzymes, proteoglycans and most recently calreticulin. Perforin (also known as cytolysin and pore-forming protein) is a 75-kDa protein that, in the presence of Ca^{2+}, polymerizes and can then insert into membranes.[27,29,30] The polyperforin then oligomerizes into a multimeric tubular structure in which the hydrophobic portions of the molecule face outward toward the cell membrane while the hydrophilic portions line the core of the tubule. These structures resemble those seen during complement-mediated lysis as a result of C9 polymerization, and are believed to correspond to the pores observed by Dourmashkin after erythrocyte ghosts were exposed to CTL.[31] Each channel consists of 12-20 perforin monomers to form a structure 16 nm high and 5-20 nm in diameter.[32] Thus a macromolecule could pass through such a channel as predicted by the mechanism, but to date only ions have actually been demonstrated to traverse.[33] Although perforin is lytic by itself, it is unable to induce DNA fragmentation within targets.[34] The genes for both human and mouse perforin have been isolated and characterized.[35,36] The sequences predict a protein of 543 amino acids, with a 20 residue leader sequence and three potential N-glycosylation sites. There is some homology with the pore-forming C9 protein of the complement cascade.

The involvement of serine proteinases in CTL and NK mediated lysis was suggested by experiments in which inhibitors of these enzymes were shown to block killing.[37,38] Two general approaches led to the identification of CTL-specific proteinases. The first was a systematic approach to identify CTL-specific mRNAs by differential screening of cDNA libraries.[39-40] Subsequent analysis using antipeptide antibodies directed against predicted protein sequences demonstrated that a number of these cytotoxic cell proteinases were localized within cytoplasmic granules.[42] Concurrently further characterization of other granule proteins led to the isolation of a number of granule proteinases.[43] The combined results of these lines of investigation have culminated in the identification of a novel family of chymotrypsin-like enzymes, most commonly referred to as granzymes. Recent experiments in which the proteins responsible for mediating DNA fragmentation (fragmentins) were identified as granzymes have confirmed the importance of these molecules in target cell lysis.[44,45] The most potent fragmentin corresponds to granzyme B (also known as CCP1). It is intriguing that this enzyme has a most unusual substrate specificity for cleavage at Asp-residues.[46] This is shared by a number of cysteine proteinases (interleukin 1 converting enzyme and ced3) that have been implicated in the induction of apoptosis in other systems.

Within the granule, the proteinases and perforin associate with chondroitin sulphate A proteoglycans.[47] Because the proteoglycans are acidic they bind tightly to basic granule proteins such as the granzymes and thus are likely involved in packaging. Chondroitin sulphate can also inhibit both perforin and proteinase activities and may serve to protect the killer cell from damage at the hands of its own lytic effectors.

GRANULE MEDIATED KILLING

Upon exocytosis the granule contents are released, possibly as a complex, and as the pH rises to neutral, active proteinases and perforin are released. The components of the granule then act in concert, in a Ca^{2+} dependent fashion, to induce lysis in the target cell. This is achieved in part by insertion of polyperforin channels in the membrane of the target cell and the induction of the apoptotic pathway by the granzymes. The perforin pores may act as channels for the passage of the granzymes and/or result in the influx of ions, such as Ca^{2+}, into the cytoplasm of the target. If we carefully consider this granule-dependent killing mechanism there are a number of stages at which calreticulin may be important. After activation the granule proteins described earlier must be transported to and sequestered in the cytoplasmic granules; could a chaperone-like molecule be involved? Prior to binding to a target cell the perforin must be maintained Ca^{2+}-free but after binding and degranulation requires a source of local Ca^{2+}. The perforin and granzymes must focus to the target cell membrane, perhaps through the involvement of an accessory molecule. Target cell lysis itself involves a Ca^{2+} influx. Could the granule-calreticulin provide such a source?

CALRETICULIN IN GRANULES

Two questions immediately arise: why doesn't calreticulin remain in the endoplasmic reticulum, and what role is a Ca^{2+}-binding protein fulfilling in cytolytic granules?

Calreticulin is normally retained in the endoplasmic reticulum by virtue of an endoplasmic reticulum retention sequence at its C-terminus. Perhaps a specific proteolytic cleavage could remove such a motif and thus release the protein from its continuous confinement in the organelle. Despite an extensive survey of monoclonal antibodies we can find no evidence for such a mechanism, i.e., the KDEL sequence is still present in granule calreticulin. Could CTL-granules represent a mini-endoplasmic reticulum in which whole portions of the larger organelle have budded off into the cytoplasm? Again this does not seem to be the case, as we are unable to demonstrate the presence of other endoplasmic reticulum-proteins (BiP, PDI, and Grp96) within the granules. Thus calreticulin localization appears to be a specific event rather than a complete suppression of the endoplasmic reticulum retention mechanism. There do appear to be two forms of calreticulin in CTL, one at 60-kDa and the other at 63-kDa, with the former being the granule-associated molecule. The basis of this difference remains unclear and possibly arises from alternate post-translational modifications. Thus, we still lack a molecular explanation for how calreticulin escapes the confines of the endoplasmic reticulum. We speculate that the KDEL retention sequence must somehow be masked, possibly by some conformational change induced by either a protein modification or through interaction with another granule protein. Clearly perforin is a likely candidate for this masking molecule but this cannot be the only explanation, as calreticulin is also found in granules from non-perforin expressing lines such as mast cells.

Let us put aside our ignorance of the explanation for how calreticulin gains entry to the granule for a moment and consider what it might be doing there. If we pause for a minute to consider that calreticulin is a Ca^{2+} binding (high and low affinity), chaperone-like (cf. calnexin) protein that can bind to integrins and influence transcriptional regulation, we seem to have an embarrassing excess of possibilities. Degranulation is Ca^{2+} dependent, perforin polymerization requires Ca^{2+} and premature exposure results in inactivation, protease activity is influenced by Ca^{2+}, and Ca^{2+} fluxes are observed in target cells under attack by CTL. We could therefore implicate calreticulin in a number of key steps in the killing process, but we believe we can exclude some of these on the basis of experimental observations. The pH of granules is around 6 and under these conditions calreticulin has a very limited ability to bind Ca^{2+}. We submit that this makes two scenarios unlikely, namely: i) calreticulin protects perforin from Ca^{2+} by acting as a Ca^{2+} buffer within the granule; ii) calreticulin is a source of "local" Ca^{2+} that allows perforin to polymerize. Clearly if calreticulin is Ca^{2+} free in the granule (this has not been formally proven) it cannot be either a source of, or a protector from, Ca^{2+} for perforin. In addition, we described earlier how CTL-mediated killing is sensitive to extracellular Ca^{2+} chelation. If calreticulin was a source of Ca^{2+} upon degranulation this result would be much less likely. Ca^{2+} independent killing has been described but appears to operate via the Fas pathway rather than the granule-dependent mechanism.[22,23]

This does not completely rule out a role for calreticulin as a Ca^{2+} binding protein in the granule-dependent killing mechanism. As perforin proceeds through the secretory pathway calreticulin could "protect" it from Ca^{2+} until it is safely sequestered within granules. During the process of degranulation, the calreticulin could once again bind Ca^{2+} and thus prevent premature polymerization of perforin.

One of the most suggestive observations concerning the role of calreticulin comes from its copurification with perforin.[17] Obviously this is a fairly tight interaction and suggests that calreticulin may indeed function as a chaperone like its cousin calnexin. Recent evidence has also indicated that this interaction is dependent upon Ca^{2+}. In the absence of Ca^{2+}, i.e. within the granule, the association is stable, whereas when Ca^{2+} is added the molecules come apart. This provides a very nice explanation for the Ca^{2+}-dependent behavior of perforin. Once dissociated from its chaperone the perforin is free to self-associate, i.e. polymerize, and insert into the target cell membrane to create transmembrane channels. It is still possible that these could provide the means of access into the target cell not only for the granzymes but also for calreticulin, where it can now influence events within its new environment. For a protein such as calreticulin, with its ability to bind cations (e.g. Ca^{2+} and Zn^{2+}) (Chapter 2) and influence the activities of other proteins, including transcription regulatory molecules and cytoskeletal elements, we have no shortage of interesting possibilities.

CONCLUDING REMARKS

In the opening paragraph we asked the question "Why should an activated immune cell need to upregulate a Ca^{2+} binding protein?" We hope that in this brief review we have convinced you that there are a number of reasons why. Many aspects of lymphocyte activation depend on precise control of Ca^{2+} levels and it is likely that calreticulin could play a role in more than one. Minimally it is likely to be a key regulator of intracytoplasmic Ca^{2+} levels after TCR engagement but its appearance in granules surely indicates a role apart in CTL-effector functioning. In our minds the most likely function is as a Ca^{2+} dependent chaperone for the lytic effector molecule perforin. However, in the absence of a direct demonstration of its action, it would be wise to keep an open mind on the function(s) of this enigmatic molecule.

ACKNOWLEDGMENTS

Work described in this review from the authors' laboratory was funded by grants from the Medical Research Council and National Cancer Institute of Canada. Robert C. Bleackley is a Medical Scientist of, and Michael J. Pinkoski holds a Studentship from, the

Alberta Heritage Foundation for Medical Research. The authors would like to thank Mae Wiley and Sherron Becker for their invaluable help in the preparation of this chapter.

REFERENCES

1. Ostwald TJ, MacLennan FH. Isolation of a high affinity Ca2+ binding protein from sarcoplasmic reticulum. Biol Chem 1974; 249:974-979.
2. Opas M, Dziak E, Fliegel L et al. Regulation of expression and intracellular distribution of calreticulin, a major Ca^{2+} binding protein of nonmuscle cells. J Cell Physiol 1991; 149:160-171.
3. Rojiani MV, Finlay BB, Gray V et al. In vitro interaction of a polypeptide homologous to human Ro/SS-A antigen (calreticulin) with a highly conserved amino acid sequence in the cytoplasmic domain of integrin alpha subunits. Biochemistry 1991; 30:9859-9865.
4. Unnasch TR, Gallin MY, Soboslay PT et al. Isolation and characterization of expression cDNA clones encoding antigens of Onchocerca volvulus infectious larvae. J Clin Invest 1988; 82:262-269.
5. Burns K, Helgason CD, Bleackley RC et al. Calreticulin in T-lymphocytes. Identification of calreticulin in T-lymphocytes and demonstration that activation of T cells correlates with increased levels of calreticulin mRNA and protein. J Biol Chem 1992; 267:19039-19042.
6. Ju S-T. Distinct pathways of CD4 and CD8 cells induce rapid target DNA fragmentation. J Immunol 1991; 146:812-818.
7. Erard F, Wild MT, Garcia-Sanz JA et al. Switch of CD8 T cells to noncytolytic CD8-CD4- cells that make TH2 cytokines and help B cells. Science 1993; 260:1802-1805.
8. Allison JP. CD28-B7 interactions in T-cell activation. Curr Opin Immunol 1994; 6:414-419.
9. Springer TA, Dustin ML, Kishimoto TK et al. The lymphocyte function-associated LFA-1, CD2, and LFA-3 molecules: Cell adhesion receptors of the immune system. Ann Rev Immunol 1987; 5:223-252.
10. Imboden J, Weiss A. The T-cell antigen receptor regulates sustained increases in cytoplasmic free Ca^{2+} through extracellular Ca^{2+} mobilization. Biochem J 1987; 247:695-700.
11. Weiss A, Imboden J, Shoback D et al. Role of T3 surface molecules in human T cell activation: T3-dependent activation results in an increase in cytoplasmic free Ca^{2+}. Proc Natl Acad Sci USA 1984; 81:4169-4173.
12. Gelfand EW. Cytosolic calcium changes during T- and B-lymphocyte activation: biological consequences and significance. Curr Top Membr Transp 1990; 35:153-177.

13. Gelfand EW, Mills GB, Cheung RK et al. Role of membrane potential in the regulation of lectin-induced calcium uptake. J Cell Physiol 1984; 122:533-539.

14. Tsien RW, Tsien RY. Ca^{2+} channels, stores and oscillations. Annu Rev Cell Biol 1990; 6:715-760.

15. Meyer T, Stryer L. Calcium spiking. Annu Rev Biophys Chem 1991; 20:153-174.

16. Clementi E, Martino G, Grimaldi LME et al. Intracellular calcium stores of T lymphocytes: changes induced by in vitro and in vivo activation. Eur J Immunol 1994; 24:1365-1371.

17. Dupuis M, Schaerer E, Krause KH et al The calcium-binding protein calreticulin is a major constituent of lytic granules in cytolytic T lymphocytes. J Exp Med 1993; 177:1-7.

18. Duke RC, Chervenak R, Cohen JJ. Endogenous endonuclease-induced DNA fragmentation: An early event in cell-mediated cytolysis. Proc Natl Acad Sci USA 1983; 80:6361-6365.

19. Berke G. The binding and lysis of target cells by cytotoxic lymphocytes: Molecular and cellular aspects. Ann Rev Immunol 1994; 12:735-773.

20. Schmid DS, Tite JP, Ruddle NH. DNA fragmentation: manifestation of target cell destruction mediated by cytotoxic T-cell lines, lymphotoxin-secreting helper T-cell clones, and cell-free lymphotoxin-containing supernatant. Proc Natl Acad Sci USA 1986; 83:1881.

21. Liu CC, Steffen M, King F et al. Identification, isolation, and characterization of novel cytotoxin in murine cytolytic lymphocytes. Cell 1987; 51:393-403.

22. Rouvier E, Lucian M-F, Golstein P. Fas involvement in Ca^{2+} independent T cell-mediated cytotoxicity. J Exp Med 1993; 177:195.

23. Garner R, Helgason CD, Atkinson EA et al. Characterization of a granule-independent lytic mechanism used by CTL hybridomas. J Immunol 1994; 53:5413-5421.

24. Kupfer A, Dennert G. Reorientation of the microtubule-organizing center and the Golgi apparatus in cloned cytotoxic lymphocytes triggered by binding to lysable target cells. J Immunol 1984; 133:2762-2766.

25. Yannelli JR, Sullivan JA, Mandell GL et al. Reorientation and fusion of cytotoxic T lymphocyte granules after interaction with target cells as determined by high resolution cinemicrography. J Immunol 1986; 136:377-382.

26. Podack ER, Kupfer A. T-cell effector functions: mechanisms for delivery of cytotoxicity and help. Ann Rev Cell Biol 1991; 7:479.

27. Henkart PA, Millard PJ, Reynolds CJ et al. Cytolytic activity of purified cytoplasmic granules from cytotoxic rat large granular lymphocyte tumors. J Exper Med 1984; 160:75-93.

28. Perry CA, Annunziato AT. Influence of histone acetylation on the solubility, H1 content and DNase I sensitivity of newly assembled chromatin. Nucleic Acids Res 1989; 17:4275-4291.

29. Masson D, Tschopp J. Isolation of a lytic, pore-forming protein (perforin) from cytolytic T-lymphocytes. J Biol Chem 1985; 260:9069-9072.

30. Podack ER, Young JDE, Cohn ZA. Isolation and biochemical and functional characterization of perforin 1 from cytolytic T-cell granules. Proc Nat Acad Sci USA 1985; 82:8629-8633.

31. Dourmashkin RR, Deteix P, Simone CB et al. Electron microscopic demonstration of lesions on target cell membranes associated with antibody-dependent cellular cytotoxicity. Clin Exp Immunol 1980; 43:554-560.

32. Tschopp J, Nabholz M. Perforin-mediated target cell lysis by cytolytic T lymphocytes. Ann Rev Immunol 1990; 8:279-302.

33. Young JD, Leong LG, Liu CC et al. Extracellular release of lymphocyte cytolytic pore-forming protein (perforin) after ionophore stimulation. Proc Natl Acad Sci USA 1986; 83:5668-5672.

34. Duke RC, Persechini PM, Chang S et al. Purified perforin induces target cell lysis but not DNA fragmentation. J Exp Med 1989; 170:1451-1456.

35. Shinkai Y, Takio K, Okumura K. Homology of perforin to the ninth component of complement (C9). Nature 1988; 334:525-527.

36. Lichtenheld MG, Olsen KJ, Lu P et al. Structure and function of human perforin. Nature 1988; 335:448-451.

37. Chang TW, Eisen HN. Effects of $N\alpha$-tosyl-L-lysyl-chloromethylketone on the activity of cytotoxic T lymphocytes. J Immunol 1980; 124:1028-1033.

38. Redelman D, Hudig D. The mechanism of cell-mediated cytotoxicity. I. Killing by murine cytotoxic T lymphocytes requires cell surface thiols and activated proteases. J Immunol 1980; 124:870.

39. Lobe CG, Finlay B, Paranchych W et al. Novel serine proteases encoded by two cytotoxic T lymphocyte-specific genes. Science 1986; 232:858-861.

40. Brunet JF, Dosseto M, Denizot F et al. The inducible cytotoxic T-lymphocyte associated gene transcript CTLA-1 sequence and gene localization to mouse chromosome 14. Nature 1986; 322:268-271.

41. Gershenfeld HK, Weissman IL. Cloning of a cDNA for a T cell-specific serine protease from a cytotoxic T lymphocyte. Science 1986; 232:854-858.

42. Redmond MJ, Lettellier M, Parker JMR et al. A serine protease (CCP1) is sequestered in the cytoplasmic granules of cytotoxic T lymphocytes. J Immunol 1987; 139:3184-3188.

43. Masson D, Tschopp J. A family of serine esterases in lytic granules of cytolytic T lymphocytes. Cell 1987; 49:679-685.

44. Shi L, Kraut RP, Aebersold R, et al. A natural killer (NK) cell granule protein that induces DNA fragmentation and apoptosis. J Exp Med 1992a; 175:553-566.

45. Shi L, Kam CM, Powers JC et al. Purification of three lymphocyte granule serine proteases that induce apoptosis through distinct substrate and target cell interactions. J Exp Med 1992b; 176:1521-1529.

46. Caputo A, James MNG, Powers JC et al. Conversion of the sub-
    strate specificity of mouse proteinase granzyme B. Nature Struc-
    tural Biology 1994; 1:364-367.
47. Stevens RL, Kamada MN, Serafin WE. Structure and function of
    the family of proteoglycans that reside in the secretory granules of
    natural killer cells and other effector cells of the immune response.
    Curr Top Microbiol Immunol 1989; 140:93-108.

CHAPTER 10

CALRETICULIN AND THROMBOSIS

David J. Pinsky, Keisuke Kuwabara, Ann Marie Schmidt,
Charles A. Lawson, Claude Benedict, Johan Broekman, Aaron
J. Marcus, Tadeusz Malinski, Jane Ryan and David M. Stern

INTRODUCTION

This chapter concerns the interaction of calreticulin with coagulation factors and vascular endothelium, as well as the anticoagulant actions of exogenously administered calreticulin. These observations[1] were quite unexpected, in that the properties of calreticulin elucidated in previous studies have pertained to its intracellular/extracellular actions unrelated to thrombosis. Calreticulin has been characterized as a ~55-kDa multifunctional Ca^{2+} binding protein which possesses three distinct structural domains; the N-domain spans the first 200 residues near the amino terminus; the P-domain (enriched in proline residues) comprises the next 131 residues; and the C-domain, containing many acidic residues, spans the carboxyl-terminal quarter of the protein (Chapter 2).[2] Although calreticulin appears to function largely as a high-capacity Ca^{2+} binding protein, there is abundant experimental data to suggest that it has other functions as well. It has recently been suggested that its localization to the endoplasmic reticulum (Chapter 3) (particularly rough endoplasmic reticulum[3]) may be the result of its putative function as a molecular chaperone, either aiding in folding of nascent polypeptides, or aiding in the retention of protein subunits prior to assembly (Chapter 4).[4] In fact, calreticulin possesses a carboxyl-terminal KDEL sequence, which acts as a retention signal for proteins destined to remain in the lumen of the endoplasmic reticulum. Although the rough endoplasmic reticulum is the preponderant location for calreticulin, it appears in some cells to also localize to the nuclear envelope,[5] and may play an active role in gene transcription (Chapter 6).[6]

Other functions have also been ascribed to calreticulin, particularly those related to immune function. Calreticulin can interact with the α-subunits of integrin receptors via a highly conserved KxGFFKR amino acid sequence present in all integrin α-subunits,[7] and may play a role in cell attachment and spreading.[8] Calreticulin and the Ca^{2+} store marker Ca^{2+}-dependent ATPase both become markedly concentrated in the filamentous actin-rich cytoplasmic area around ingested particles during phagocytosis in neutrophils, suggesting that calreticulin may play a role in highly localized increases in intracellular Ca^{2+}, which may be of functional significance.[9] In addition, several studies have suggested that calreticulin plays a role in T cell activation; activation of T cells correlates with increased levels of calreticulin mRNA and protein,[10] and calreticulin is a major constituent of lytic granules in cytolytic T lymphocytes,[11] where it may prevent perforin-mediated autolysis due to its Ca^{2+}-chelating ability (Chapter 8).

ISOLATION OF CALRETICULIN BASED UPON ITS ABILITY TO BIND FACTOR IX

Calreticulin was identified fortuitously by Kuwabara et al[1] in a series of experiments designed to isolate polypeptides which bind to the vitamin K-dependent coagulation factor, Factor IX. There were a number of important reasons behind the undertaking to isolate and characterize polypeptides which bind to Factor IX. Factor IXa may contribute to the pathogenesis of thrombosis,[12-14] and it is rapidly bound to both platelets and endothelium.[15-17] To isolate endothelial proteins with putative Factor IX binding sites, bovine lung tissue was used as a starting material because of the rich vasculature and abundant endothelium of the lungs, an approach which had been used with previous success for purifying endothelial cell receptors.[18,19] Lung extracts were immobilized on polyvinyl chloride wells, and specific binding of ^{125}I-Factor IX was evaluated. Binding of ^{125}I-Factor IX to immobilized lung extracts occurred in a dose-dependent fashion, with a K_d ~1.6 nM (close to the reported affinity of Factor IX to endothelial cells and platelets[16,17]). However, this binding was not specific, for prothrombin and Factor X also competed with Factor IX for binding sites in lung extracts.

To further characterize the polypeptides in the lung extract which bound Factor IX, the material was subjected to a series of chromatographic steps, including hydroxylapatite and FPLC Mono Q chromatography, and eluted fractions were tested for Factor IX binding activity following adsorption to microtiter wells (Fig. 10.1). SDS-PAGE demonstrated a single band with an M_r of ~55,000 to be closely associated with Factor IX binding activity. Elution of this ~55-kDa protein was followed by amino-terminal sequencing, as well as sequencing of several fragments following tryptic digestion, which revealed significant sequence homology with calreticulin from several species, including rabbit, dog, rat, pig, and human.[20-24]

Based upon this sequence data, identifying the Factor IX-binding protein as calreticulin, further experiments were performed with purified recombinant rabbit calreticulin[25] to test both its binding to vitamin K-dependent coagulation factors, as well as its potential in vitro and in vivo anticoagulant functions. In addition to comigrating on SDS-PAGE with the 55-kDa band isolated from

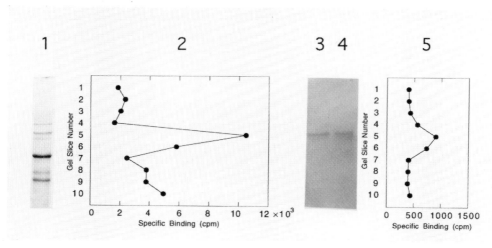

Fig. 10.1. SDS-PAGE and gel elution of the ~55-kDa polypeptide derived from lung extract which binds factor IX. **1.** Coomassie Blue staining of a nonreduced SDS-PAGE of the pool from the FPLC Mono Q column with Factor IX binding activity. **2.** Factor IX binding activity profile of material shown in panel 1. **3.** Silver-stained reduced gel of material eluted from slices 5 and 6 in panel 2. **4.** Same as in panel 3, but with nonreduced gel. **5.** Factor IX-binding activity profile of material eluted from gel shown in panel 4. Adapted from Kuwabara K, Pinsky DJ, Schmidt AM et al. J Biol Chem 1995; 270:8179-8187.

bovine lung, recombinant calreticulin was shown to possess similar binding characteristics for other vitamin K-dependent coagulation factors; half-maximal binding by recombinant calreticulin for Factors IX, X, and prothrombin was observed at 2.7, 3.2, and 8.3 nM, respectively (Fig. 10.2). Furthermore, competition experiments showed that these vitamin K-dependent coagulation factors competed with each other for binding, suggesting that they interacted with identical or overlapping sites on calreticulin.

Further experiments revealed that the interaction of calreticulin with ^{125}I-Factor IX was Ca^{2+}-dependent. Because calreticulin possesses three functional domains (N, P, and C domains (Chapter 2)), the next series of experiments was performed to determine

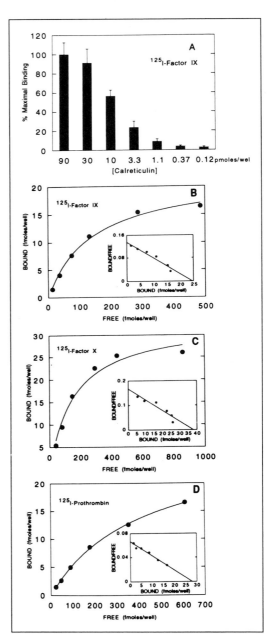

Fig. 10.2. Binding of Factors IX, X, and prothrombin to recombinant purified rabbit calreticulin. **A.** Microtiter wells were coated with the indicated concentrations of calreticulin and the specific binding of ^{125}I-labeled Factor IX was measured. **B-D.** Microtiter wells were coated with 9.2 pmol/well of calreticulin, and specific binding of the indicated factors measured in the presence and absence of 100-fold molar excess of the unlabelled respective proteins. Specific binding is plotted versus the free/added concentration of ^{125}I-labeled clotting factor. Adapted from Kuwabara K, Pinsky DJ, Schmidt AM et al. J Biol Chem 1995; 270:8179-8187.

which of the three domains was responsible for Factor IX binding. These experiments demonstrated that only the low affinity/high capacity Ca^{2+} binding domain (the C domain) was responsible for factor IX binding activity. Not surprisingly, similar experiments demonstrated that the C domain also possessed factor X and prothrombin binding activity, whereas the other domains did not.

EFFECT OF CALRETICULIN ON VITAMIN K-DEPENDENT COAGULANT FUNCTION

Because calreticulin interacts with multiple coagulation factors, experiments were performed to determine whether calreticulin affects coagulation reactions in vitro. To determine the effect of calreticulin on the extrinsic coagulation pathway, in which tissue factor interacts with Factor VIIa to activate Factor X, leading to the sequential conversions of prothrombin to thrombin and fibrinogen to fibrin, the effect of calreticulin on tissue factor VIIa/Factor VIIa-mediated activation of factor X was studied. These experiments used tissue factor prepared from tumor necrosis factor-treated endothelial cell matrices, as previously reported.[26] Calreticulin did not alter Factor Xa formation, regardless of the concentration used, indicating lack of antithrombotic effect at the level of Factor VIIa/tissue factor. Similarly, calreticulin did not alter Factor Xa/Va-mediated activation of prothrombin, and had no effect on the clotting time initiated by thromboplastin. These studies demonstrate that calreticulin does not affect the extrinsic or final common coagulation pathway of coagulation in vitro.

Experiments were then performed to determine whether calreticulin might affect the intrinsic coagulation pathway in vitro, which would not be surprising given its avid binding to vitamin K-dependent coagulation factors. Calreticulin was used over a wide range of concentrations for the following experiments, in which Factor Xa formation and clotting times were measured under standardized conditions in vitro using cephalin or endothelium as the phospholipid surface upon which reaction could occur. Neither Factor IXa-VIIIa-mediated activation of Factor X nor the clotting time of plasma initiated by addition of Factor IXa were altered in the presence of calreticulin. These studies demonstrate that calreticulin does not affect the intrinsic coagulation pathway in vitro.

To investigate whether calreticulin might have an effect on the vitamin K-dependent, endothelium-based, protein C anticoagulant pathway, the effect of calreticulin on thrombinthrombomodulin-mediated formation of activated protein C was studied. This pathway utilizes thrombomodulin, a transmembrane protein expressed by endothelium, which accelerates the conversion of the zymogen protein C to the enzyme activated protein C by thrombin.[18] The effect of calreticulin on this pathway was investigated using intact bovine endothelial cells as the source of thrombomodulin. In the presence of thrombin, thrombomodulin, and protein C, the rate of release of p-nitroanilide (formed by activated protein C-mediated hydrolysis of the chromogenic substrate Lys-Pro-Arg-p-nitroanilide) is monitored.[27,28] Calreticulin had no effect on this reaction, suggesting that it does not impair or augment thrombomodulin-dependent, thrombin-mediated activation of protein C. Thus, although calreticulin binds to multiple vitamin K-dependent coagulation factors, it does not appear to directly alter their coagulant properties based on our studies with purified coagulation components in vitro.

IN VIVO ANTITHROMBOTIC EFFECTS OF CALRETICULIN

To establish if calreticulin affected the coagulation mechanism in vivo, the effects of calreticulin were studied in an in vivo canine coronary thrombosis model. In this model,[14,29] an electric current was delivered intraluminally to the left circumflex coronary artery until a 50% decrease in cross-sectional area was achieved (measured based upon the inverse relation between cross-sectional area and flow velocity measured using a doppler flow probe). After this initial thrombogenic event, current was discontinued, and either saline or calreticulin was given as an intracoronary bolus. Over the ensuing three hour observation period, all saline treated dogs developed progressive (occlusive) thrombosis, whereas dogs treated with the maximal dose of calreticulin (1.2 mg/animal) did not develop coronary occlusion (Fig. 10.3). Dose-response experiments demonstrated that the in vivo antithrombotic effects of calreticulin were roughly proportional to the infused dose, with no effect observed with the lowest dose studied (200 µg/animal). As predicted from the in vitro coagulation studies which failed to demonstrate an effect of calreticulin on plasma clotting times, both the activated partial thromboplastin time and prothrombin time were not affected by intracoronary infusion of calreticulin. Since calreticulin had no direct effect on properties of soluble coagulation components, our attention was directed to its potential interaction with the vessel wall.

CALRETICULIN INTERACTIONS WITH VASCULAR ENDOTHELIUM

Investigations were undertaken to determine how calreticulin might interact with the cells forming the luminal vascular surface, the endothelium. Binding studies were performed with confluent monolayers of bovine aortic endothelial cells, using ^{125}I-labeled calreticulin. These studies demonstrated that ^{125}I-calreticulin bound to endothelial cells in a reversible manner, depending on the dose of radioligand (K_d ~7.4 nM; Fig. 10.4). The endothelial binding site(s) for calreticulin are likely to be distinct from those for Factor IX, because excess unlabeled calreticulin did not alter the

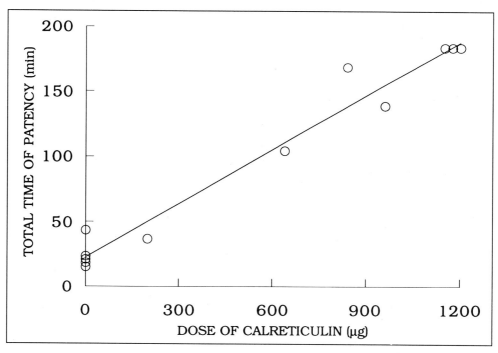

Fig. 10.3. Antithrombotic effect of intracoronary calreticulin in a canine electrically-induced left circumflex coronary artery thrombosis model. Following an initial application of current to incite 50% luminal thrombosis, the time until complete occlusion is shown following the intracoronary administration of the indicated concentrations of calreticulin. Adapted from Kuwabara K, Pinsky DJ, Schmidt AM et al. J Biol Chem 1995; 270:8179-8187.

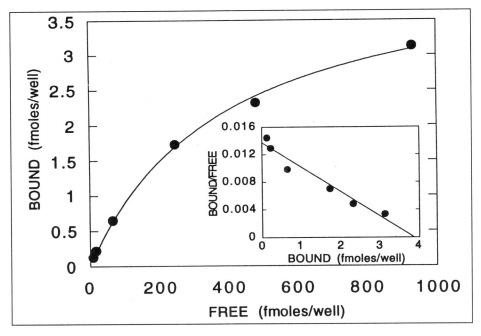

Fig. 10.4A

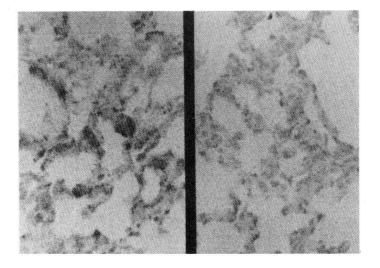

Fig. 10.4B

*Fig. 10.4. Binding of calreticulin to endothelial cells. **A.** Confluent monolayers of bovine aortic endothelial cells were incubated with the indicated concentration of ^{125}I-calreticulin alone or in the presence of a 100-fold molar excess of the unlabeled protein. Specific binding is plotted versus the free/added concentration of ^{125}I-calreticulin. K_d ~7.4 nM. **B.** Immuno-histochemical localization of recombinant rabbit calreticulin following tail vein infusion in mice. Left panel demonstrates vascular staining (lung tissue is shown) following calreticulin infusion, whereas the right panel fails to demonstrate similar staining following infusion of a control protein (albumin). Adapted from Kuwabara K, Pinsky DJ, Schmidt AM et al. J Biol Chem 1995; 270:8179-8187.*

binding of radiolabelled Factor IX, nor did antibody to calreticulin alter the binding of Factor IX to endothelial cells.

In vivo studies performed by infusing recombinant calreticulin into mice confirmed the in vitro endothelial binding studies demonstrating endothelial binding of calreticulin. Infused calreticulin was rapidly cleared from the circulation (Fig. 10.5), and found to be associated prominently with the endothelium in most vascular organs, particularly the lungs (Fig. 10.4B).

To determine whether calreticulin might influence endothelial properties relevant to coagulation, the effects of calreticulin on endothelial nitric oxide (NO) production were studied. NO, also known as endothelium-derived relaxing factor, is a powerful inhibitor of platelet aggregation.[30] Under basal conditions, it is formed in endothelial cells from the amino acid L-arginine by the constitutive isoform of NO synthase, an effect which is triggered by brief Ca^{2+} transients within the endothelial cell. This is often a receptor mediated event, and a number of agonists, such as thrombin, histamine, bradykinin, or acetylcholine, may trigger bursts of NO synthesis. The effects of calreticulin on endothelial NO synthesis were studied in two ways. Direct measurements of NO synthesis were performed using a porphyrinic microsensor as a specific and sensitive way to study the kinetic release of NO[31-33] in response to applied calreticulin. These studies demonstrated that calreticulin had a dose-dependent effect to increase endothelial NO

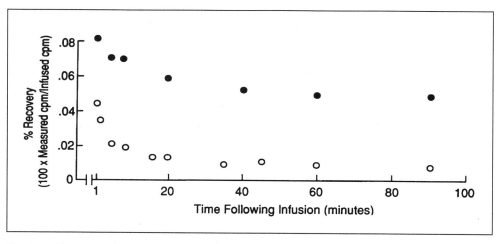

Fig. 10.5. Clearance of exogenously administered thrombomodulin. Mice were given an intravenous injection of either ^{125}I-labeled recombinant rabbit calreticulin (○) or a similar dose of ^{125}I-albumin (●) as a control. Calreticulin clearance is rapid and early in comparison with the control protein. Adapted from Kuwabara K, Pinsky DJ, Schmidt AM et al. J Biol Chem 1995; 270:8179-8187.

production (approximately 14 ± 2 fmol of NO/s/1 nM calreticulin), that was not seen with similar applications of a control protein such as albumin (Fig. 10.6). The concentrations of calreticulin required to induce NO release from endothelial cells were comparable to those concentrations of calreticulin required for binding to endothelial cells.

To further explore the relevance of calreticulin-induced NO production for potential antithrombotic effects, the effects of calreticulin to induce NO synthesis were measured in a bioassay which measures endothelial cell-derived NO based on its ability to inhibit platelet aggregation and serotonin release in response to a thrombin challenge.[32,34] These studies showed that, in the presence of endothelial cells, calreticulin inhibited both thrombin-mediated platelet aggregation, as well as serotonin release. Because this effect was inhibited by the application of hemoglobin, which binds to NO to inactivate its biological effects, these studies confirm

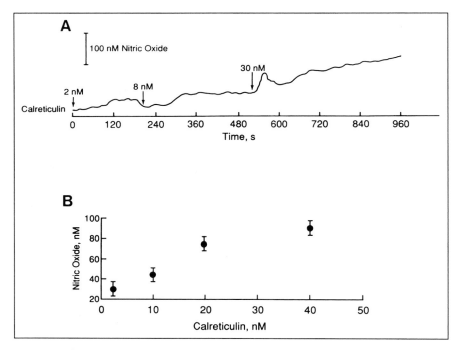

Fig. 10.6. Effect of calreticulin to increase endothelial nitric oxide production. Nitric oxide levels were measured using a porphyrinic microsensor. **A.** Chronoamperometric recordings of NO produced by bovine aortic endothelial cell monolayers are shown, with the indicated concentrations of calreticulin applied in the bathing solution in which the recordings were made. **B.** Nitric oxide levels measured at the endothelial surface as a function of applied calreticulin concentration. Adapted from Kuwabara K, Pinsky DJ, Schmidt AM et al. J Biol Chem 1995; 270:8179-8187.

that calreticulin appears to inhibit platelet aggregation by its effects to increase endothelial NO production.

These findings are particularly interesting, in light of the work by Liu et al,[35] in a neuroblastoma/glioma cell line; reducing calreticulin (using an antisense oligodeoxynucleotide) interferes with Ca^{2+} transients evoked by inositol 1,4,5-trisphosphate synthesis in response to bradykinin. Preliminary studies from our lab have suggested that localized Ca^{2+} transients may also occur in endothelial cells exposed to exogenous calreticulin, perhaps explaining the immediate and sustained increase in endothelial NO synthesis which we have observed following application of calreticulin. When the results of in vitro endothelial binding studies, in vivo clearance studies with immunohistochemical localization to the vascular wall, and NO studies are considered together, these data suggest that calreticulin may act as an antithrombotic agent by promoting localized, endogenous, NO-dependent antithrombotic mechanisms.

SUMMARY

Calreticulin, identified in lung extracts based upon its ability to bind to Factor IX, was found to similarly bind to other vitamin K-dependent coagulation factors (II and X) via its C-domain. Although binding of calreticulin to lung extracts was specific and saturable, binding sites for calreticulin appeared to be distinct from those for the vitamin K-dependent coagulation factors. Cross-competition studies demonstrated that although the binding of vitamin K-dependent coagulation factors to calreticulin was dose-dependent and saturable, this binding appeared to result from interaction with the same or overlapping sites on calreticulin. In vitro and in vivo studies demonstrated that calreticulin had no direct effect on the intrinsic or extrinsic coagulation pathways, nor did it alter thrombin/thrombomodulin-mediated activation of protein C. Binding studies demonstrated a high affinity binding site for calreticulin on endothelial cells (K_d ~7.4 nM), and infusion studies demonstrated rapid localization of calreticulin to the vascular wall. Direct intracoronary administration of calreticulin was associated with a dose-dependent inhibition of coronary thrombosis in an electrically-induced canine coronary artery thrombosis model, without affecting systemic coagulant function. Further endothelium-based studies performed to determine the nature of the calreticulin-induced anticoagulant mechanism showed that calreticulin caused a dose-dependent, immediate, and sustained release of nitric oxide from endothelial cells. As nitric oxide so produced was a potent inhibitor of platelet aggregation and serotonin release, these studies suggest that, following infusion, calreticulin may stimulate local production of endothelium-derived nitric oxide, providing a basis for its anticoagulant properties.

REFERENCES

1. Kuwabara K, Pinsky DJ, Schmidt AM et al. Calreticulin, an antithrombotic agent which binds to vitamin K-dependent coagulation factors, stimulates endothelial nitric oxide production, and limits thrombosis in canine coronary arteries. J Biol Chem 1995; 270:8179-8187.
2. Baksh S, Michalak M. Expression of calreticulin in *Escherichia coli* and identification of its Ca^{2+} binding domains. J Biol Chem 1991; 266:21458-21465.
3. Tharin S, Dziak E, Michalak M et al. Widespread tissue distribution of rabbit calreticulin, a non-muscle functional analogue of calsequestrin. Cell Tissue Res 1992; 269:29-37.
4. Nigam SK, Goldberg AL, Ho S et al. A set of endoplasmic reticulum proteins possessing properties of molecular chaperones includes Ca^{2+}-binding proteins and members of the thioredoxin superfamily. J Biol Chem 1994; 269:1744-1749.
5. Opas M, Dziak E, Fliegel L et al. Regulation of expression and intracellular distribution of calreticulin, a major calcium binding protein of nonmuscle cells. J Cell Physiol 1991; 149160-171.
6. Burns K, Duggan B, Atkinson EA et al. Modulation of gene expression by calreticulin binding to the glucocorticoid receptor. Nature 1994; 67:476-480.
7. Rojiani MV, Finlay BB, Gray V et al. In vitro interaction of a polypeptide homologous to human Ro/SS-A antigen (calreticulin) with a highly conserved amino acid sequence in the cytoplasmic domain of integrin alpha subunits. Biochemistry 1991; 30:9859-98661.
8. Leung-Hagesteijn CY, Milankov K, Michalak M et al. Cell attachment to extracellular matrix substrates is inhibited upon downregulation of expression of calreticulin, an intracellular integrin α-subunit-binding protein. J Cell Sci 1994; 107:589-600.
9. Stendahl O, Krause K-H, Krischer J et al. Redistribution of intracellular Ca^{2+} stores during phagocytosis in human neutrophils. Science 1994; 265:1439-1441.
10. Burns K, Helgason CD, Bleackley RC et al. Calreticulin in T-lymphocytes. Identification of calreticulin in T-lymphocytes and demonstration that activation of T cells correlates with increased levels of calreticulin mRNA and protein. J Biol Chem 1992; 267:19039-19042.

11. Dupuis M, Schaerer E, Krause K-H et al. The calcium-binding protein calreticulin is a major constituent of lytic granules in cytolytic T lymphocytes. J Exp Med 1993; 177:1-7.

12. Gurewich V, Nunn T, Lipinski B. Activation of intrinsic or extrinsic blood coagulation in experimental venous thrombosis and disseminated intravascular coagulation: pathogenetic differences. Thromb Res 1979; 14:931-940.

13. Gitel SN, Stephenson RC, Wessler S. In vitro and in vivo correlation of clotting protease activity: effect of heparin. Proc Natl Acad Sci USA 1977; 74:3028-3032.

14. Benedict CR, Ryan J, Wolitzky B et al. Active site-blocked factor IXa prevents intravascular thrombus formation in the coronary vasculature without inhibiting extravascular coagulation in a canine thrombosis model. J Clin Invest 1991; 88:1760-1765.

15. Heimark RL, Schwartz SM. Binding of coagulation factors IX and X to the endothelial cell surface. Biochem Biophys Res Commun 1983; 111:723-731.

16. Stern DM, Drillings M, Nossel J et al. Activation of factor IX bound to cultured bovine aortic endothelial cells. Proc Natl Acad Sci USA 1993; 81:913-917.

17. Ahmad SS, Rawala-Sheikh R, Ashby B et al. Platelet receptor-mediated factor X activation by factor IXa. High-affinity factor IXa receptors induced by factor VIII are deficient on platelets in Scott syndrome. J Clin Invest 1989; 84:824-828.

18. Esmon NL, Owen WG, Esmon CT. Isolation of a membrane-bound cofactor for thrombin-catalyzed activation of protein C. J Biol Chem 1982; 257:859-864.

19. Schmidt AM, Vianna M, Gerlach M et al. Isolation and characterization of binding proteins for advanced glycosylation end products from lung tissue which are present on the endothelial cell surface. J Biol Chem 1992; 267:14987-14997.

20. Collins JH, Xi ZJ, Alderson-Lang BH et al. Sequence homology of a canine brain calcium-binding protein with calregulin and the human Ro/SS-A antigen. Biochem Biophys Res Commun 1989; 164:575-579.

21. Fliegel L, Burns K, MacLennan DH et al. Molecular cloning of the high affinity calcium-binding protein (calreticulin) of skeletal muscle sarcoplasmic reticulum. J Biol Chem 1989; 264:21522-21528.

22. Van PN, Peter F, Söling H-D. Four intracisternal calcium-binding glycoproteins from rat liver microsomes with high affinity for calcium. No indication for calsequestrin-like proteins in inositol 1,4,5-trisphosphate-sensitive calcium sequestering rat liver vesicles. J Biol Chem 1989; 264:17494-17501.

23. Rokeach L, Haselby J, Meilof J et al. Characterization of the autoantigen calreticulin. J Immunol 1991; 147:3031-3039.

24. Milner R, Baksh S, Shemanko C et al. Calreticulin, and not calsequestrin, is the major calcium binding protein of smooth muscle sarcoplasmic reticulum and liver endoplasmic reticulum. J Biol Chem 1991; 266:7155-7165.

25. Baksh S, Burns K, Busaan J et al. Expression and purification of recombinant and native calreticulin. Prot Exp Pur 1992; 3:322-331.

26. Ryan J, Brett J, Tijburg P et al. Tumor necrosis factor-induced endothelial tissue factor is associated with subendothelial matrix vesicles but is not expressed on the apical surface. Blood 1992; 80:966-974.

27. Nawroth P, Stern DM. Modulation of endothelial cell homeostatic properties by tumor necrosis factor. J Exp Med 1986; 163:740-745.

28. Koga S, Morris S, Ogawa S et al. TNF modulates endothelial permeability and anticoagulant properties by activating phosphodiesterase and decreasing cAMP. Am J Physiol 1995; 268: C1104-C1113.

29. Benedict CR, Mathew B, Rex KA et al. Correlation of plasma serotonin changes with platelet aggregation in an in vivo dog model of spontaneous occlusive coronary thrombus formation. Circ Res 1986; 73:58-67.

30. Lowenstein C, Snyder S. Nitric oxide, a novel biologic messenger. Cell 1992; 70:705-707.

31. Malinski T, Taha Z. Nitric oxide release from a single cell measured in situ by a porphyrinic-based microsensor. Nature 1992; 358: 676-678.

32. Pinsky DJ, Naka Y, Chowdhury NC et al. The nitric oxide/cyclic GMP pathway in organ transplantation: critical role in successful lung preservation, Proc Natl Acad Sci USA 1994; 91:12086-120904.

33. Pinsky DJ, Oz MC, Koga S et al. Cardiac preservation is enhanced in a heterotopic rat transplant model by supplementing the nitric oxide pathway. J Clin Invest 1994; 93:2291-2297.

34. Broekman M, Eiroa A, Marcus A. Inhibition of human platelet reactivity by endothelium-derived relaxing factor from human umbilical vein endothelial cells in suspension. Blood 1991; 78:1033-1040.

35. Liu N, Fine RE, Simons E et al. Decreasing calreticulin expression lowers the Ca^{2+} response to bradykinin and increases sensitivity to ionomycin in NG-108-15 cells. J Biol Chem 1994; 269:28635-28639.

CHAPTER 11

CALRETICULIN IN VECTOR ARTHROPODS—THE SECRETED CALRETICULIN

Deborah C. Jaworski and Glen R. Needham

INTRODUCTION

One of the most unusual places calreticulin has been found is the saliva of ticks.[1] Most calreticulins are located intracellularly. Our work objective was to characterize and clone salivary secretions that induce host immunity to tick feeding.[2,3] Host immune response to tick feeding was demonstrated in domesticated animals as early as 1918.[4] Trager[5] experimentally documented host resistance to tick feeding. Using host immune sera in Western blots, we began to characterize antigens expressed and secreted during the first six days of feeding. Through our tick salivary gland cDNA library and these host immune sera, we discovered that a major gland secretion is calreticulin.[1]

Host immune responses in ticks are modulated by the salivary glands (Fig. 11.1). The salivary glands in the tick extend from the "head" back two-thirds the length of its body, contain three different acinar types and undergo a dramatic morphogenesis during a long feeding interval (up to 3 weeks).[6] Tick salivary secretions produced during feeding contain a variety of components that can modulate events at the attachment site including the transmission of pathogens.[7-11] Sonenshine[12] lists many of the substances that have been found in the tick salivary glands. While some components of salivary secretions have been identified, none have been fully characterized.[13-17] The specific impact of any one component in the feeding lesion has been difficult to determine due to the small amounts of saliva or salivary gland tissue. Unlike many of the other calreticulins reported in this volume, the significance of calreticulin in ticks and other blood feeding arthropods is just now being studied.

TICKS AND CALRETICULIN

We performed immuno-screening of a salivary gland cDNA expression library prepared from fed lone star ticks (*Amblyomma americanum* females). A polyspecific antiserum to 3-day feeding salivary gland extracts was used.[2] We previously determined that

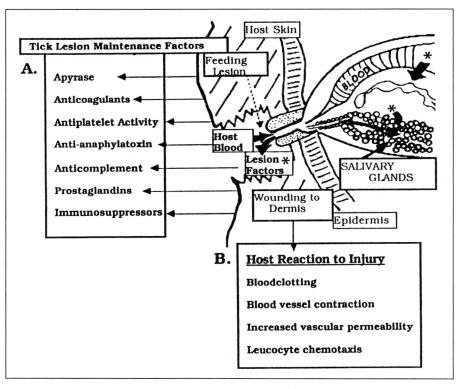

Fig. 11.1. Diagrammatic representation of the dynamic relationship between an ixodid tick and its host (adapted from G.R. Needham, unpublished). Salivary glands gain competence to secrete soon after attachment to the host. Panel **A** represents some of the many factors that a tick secretes into the feeding lesion. These factors counteract the host response to injury (panel **B**), and maintain the feeding lesion over a period of days to several weeks until the tick fully engorges and drops from the host. The long feeding interval provides ample time for tick-borne pathogens to be mobilized and injected with these secreted factors.

this antiserum recognizes gland polypeptides that are feeding-specific. Here, we summarize our research on the cloned salivary gland protein, 161A, which is homologous to the Ca^{2+}-binding protein, calreticulin. This protein appears to be secreted during the feeding process and is detected in dopamine/theophylline-stimulated saliva. Further details about the methods and results are presented elsewhere.[1]

To characterize 161A in the salivary glands during tick feeding, we first prepared an antibody to 161A. The fusion protein was immobilized on nitrocellulose membrane, excised and directly implanted into a New Zealand White rabbit. The resulting polyclonal antibody detects a single band in our fusion protein extract, and in purified rabbit skeletal muscle calreticulin. Protein 161A was evident in salivary glands during feeding, but was in low abundance in non-feeding females. Protein 161A was most evident in the salivary glands of ticks fed 3 and 6 days. In midgut tissues, 161A was only observed after 6 days of feeding. When ticks were fed on rabbits immunized with 161A-fusion protein, the feeding sites were necrotic and hemorrhagic with visible cavities in the epidermis (Fig. 11.2). This local host response was very different from that of non-immunized hosts where overt bite-site reaction is usually not observed (Fig. 11.3). One explanation is that antibody to the fusion protein binds calreticulin, thereby initiating a localized immune reaction to tick infestation. The immune reaction may disrupt the feeding cycle; however, ticks fed on the immunized host fed normally, gained weights equal to controls and laid egg masses similar to controls. These data indicate that 161A is synthesized and secreted into the host during the tick feeding interval.

Amino acid sequence for 161A is shown (Fig. 11.4). Clone 161A is over 69% homologous to rabbit skeletal muscle calreticulin.[18] These two amino acid sequences are more than 80% homologous in the N-terminal domain; and 41% homologous in the C-terminal region. Molecular mass for tick calreticulin was 58-kDa and within the range of reported values for calreticulins, 55-63-kDa, as measured by migration in SDS-polyacrylamide gels.[19] A major difference between 161A and other calreticulins is the lack of an endoplasmic reticulum retention signal KDEL—161A ends with HEEL. Two putative Ca^{2+}-binding regions have been identified in rabbit skeletal muscle calreticulin.[19] The high affinity, low capacity region in the P-domain is retained in the secreted tick calreticulin. The C-terminal domain is quite different for the tick; however, acidic residues predominate and a Ca^{2+}-binding function could be retained. On the basis of our immune sera screening results, the missing KDEL sequence, and its presence in the saliva of two tick species, 161A represents a calreticulin that is routed through a secretory pathway rather than being retained in the endoplasmic reticulum.

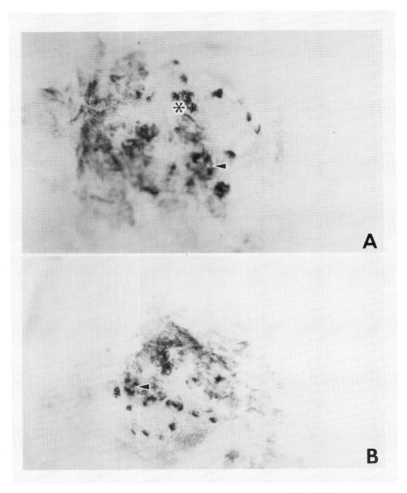

*Fig. 11.2. Feeding lesion observed on rabbit immunized with fusion protein 161A. Feeding lesion observed on this rabbit was atypical of a first infestation response to tick feeding. Panel **A**. Arrow indicates one area of necrosis and bleeding at the bite site. Other areas were also affected. Some of the male ticks, still attached when all the females had dropped, are indicated by the asterisk. Panel **B**. Lower magnification of lesion shown in Panel **A**.*

We used immunoblots to confirm that 161A is calreticulin, and to determine whether it is a secreted protein in ticks. Authentic antibody to purified rabbit calreticulin reacts with a 58-kDa protein in tick salivary glands and the 64-kDa polypeptide fusion protein from clone 161A. Calreticulin was identified in the saliva and migrated to a similar position as purified calreticulin in side-by-side gel lanes. Calreticulin was present in the saliva of both *A. americanum* and *Dermacentor variabilis*. A constitutive form of calreticulin should also exist in ticks, although this is yet

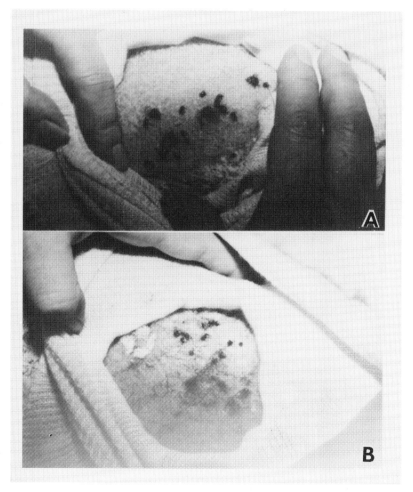

Fig. 11.3. Typical feeding lesion seen on naive and resistant host. Panel **A**. Feeding lesion on naive host. Bite sites slightly raised with slight erythema. Panel **B**. Feeding lesion on resistant host (after four infestations). Bite sites with edema, erythema and visible serous exudate.

Calreticulin Homologies (Modified from Michalak et al. 1992)

```
            10          20          30          40          50          60          70          80
Rabbit    EPVVYFKEQF  LDGDGWTERW  IESKHKSDFG  KFVLSSGKFY  GDQEKDKGLQ  TSQDARFYAL  SARFEPFSNK  GQPLVVQFTV
Human     EPAVYFKEQF  LDGDGWTSRW  IESKHKSDFG  KFVLSSGKFY  GDEEKDKGLQ  TSQDARFYAL  SASFE-FSNK  GQPTVVQFTV
RAL-1     NAKIYFKEDF  SDDD-WEKRW  IKSKHKDDFG  K--WIEGKFY  GDAVKDKGLK  TTQDAKFYSI  CAKFDKSSNK  GQKSVVIFTS
Sm4       GHEVWFSETF  PNESIENWVQ  STYNAEKQGE  FKVEAGKSPV  DPIEDLGLKT  TTQDARFYGI  ARKISETFSNR GKTMVLQFTV
Tick 161A  Incomplete NH2 - end                          GTSAGKFY    GDAEKSKGLQ  TSEDARFYGI  SSKFEPFSNE  GKTL-WQFTV

            90         100         110         120         130         140         150         160
Rabbit    KHEQNIDCGG  GYVKLFPAGL  DQKDMHGDSE  YNIMFGPDIC  GPGTKKVHVI  FNYKGKNVLI  NKDIRCKDDE  FTHLYTLIVR
Human     KHEQNIDCGG  GYVKLFPNSL  DQTDMHGDSE  YNIMFGPDIC  GPGTKKVHVI  FNYKGKNVLI  NKDIRCKDDE  FTHLYTLIVR
RAL-1     KHEQNDDCGG  GYVKLMASDV  NLEDSHGETP  YHIMFGPDIC  GPGTKKVHVI  FHYKDRNHMI  KKDIRCKDDV  FTHIYTLIVN
Sm4       KFDKTVSCGG  AYIKLLGSDI  DPKKFHGESP  YRIMFGPDIC  GMATKKVHVI  FNYKGKNHLI  KKEIPCKDDL  KTHLYTLIVN
Tick 161A KHEQNIDCGG  GYVKLFDCSL  DQTQMHGESP  YKIMFGPDIC  GPGTKKVHVI  FNYKGKNHLI  NKEIRCKDDY  FTHLYTLIVK

           170         180         190         200         210         220         230         240
Rabbit    PDNTYEVKID  NSQVESGSLE  DDWDFLPPKK  IKDPDASKPE  DWDERAKIDD  PTDSKPEDWD  KPEHIPDPDA  KKPEDWDEEM
Human     PDNTYEVKID  NSQVESGSLE  DDWDFLPPKK  IKDPDASKPE  DWDERAKIDD  PTDSKPEDWD  KPEHIPDPDA  KKPEDWDEEM
RAL-1     SDNTYFVQID  GFKAESGELE  ADWDFLPPKK  IKDPDAKKPE  DWDEREFIDD  EDDKKPEDWD  KPEHIPDPDA  KKPEDWDDEM
Sm4       PNNKYEVLVD  NAKVEEGSLE  DDWDMLPPKK  IDDPNDKKPD  DWVDEQFIDD  PDDKKPDNWD  QPKTIPDNDA  KKPDDWDDDAM
Tick 161A PDNTYVVKID  NEVAEKGELE  SDWSFLPPKK  IKDPEAKKPE  DWDDRAKIDD  PEDKKPEDWD  KPEYIPDPDA  TKPEDWDDDM

           250         260         270         280         290         300         310         320
Rabbit    DGEWEPPVIQ  NPEYKGEWKP  RQIDNPDYKG  TWIHPEIDNP  EYSPDANIYA  YDSFAVLGLD  LWQVLSGTIF  DNFLITNDEA
Human     DGEWEPPVIQ  NPEYKGEWKP  PQIDNPDYKG  TWIHPEIDNP  EYSPDPDIYA  YDNFGVLGLD  LWQVKSGTIF  DNFLITNDEA
RAL-1     DGEWEPPMVD  NPEYKGEWKP  KQKKNPAWKG  KWHPEIEIP   DYTPDDNLYV  YDDIGAIGFD  LWQVLSGTIF  DDVIVTDSVE
Sm4       DGEWERPQKD  NPEYKGEWTP  RRIDNPKYKG  EWKPVQIDNP  EYKHDPELYV  LNDIGYVGFD  LWQVDSGSIF  DNILTDSPD
Tick 161A DGEWEPPQIN  NPEYKGEWKP  KQIDNPAYKG  AWVHPEIDNP  EYTADPKLYH  FPELCTIGFD  LWQVKSGTIF  DNLLTDDEE

           330         340         350         360         370         380         390         401
Rabbit    YAEEFGNETW  GVTKTAEKZM  KDKQDEEQRL  KEEEEEKKRK  EEEEAEEDEE  DKDDKEDEKE  DEEDKDEEEE  EAAAGQAKDEL
Human     YAEEFGNETW  GVTKTAEKZM  KDKQDEEQRL  KEEEEEKKRK  EEEEAEDKED  K-EEKDEDEE  DEEDKDEEEE  EDVPGQAKDEL
RAL-1     EAKKFGEKTL  KKIKREGKQ-  KD----GQKT  ------KKRK  -EKENEKIK   EKMKKRKRAN  R - KKKK
Sm4       FAKEEGERLW  RKRYDAEVAK  EQSSAKDDK   EAAEETKERK  ELPYDAKCDD  PSGDHDEL
Tick 161A YARVHGEETW  AALKDEEKM   KEKQEEEDA   KSKKEDDAKD  EDEFEDEEET  EDKEKEDEET  TAAPEDDHK   HEEL
```

undetermined. Physiological roles for calreticulin are still unknown, and its presence in tick saliva suggests an extracellular role for this protein. In the absence of experimental evidence, we take this opportunity to explore some potential roles for calreticulin in ticks and other blood sucking arthropods.

ROLE OF CALRETICULIN IN TICKS/BLOOD FEEDING ARTHROPODS

Roles of Ca^{2+} in controlling fluid secretion in ixodid ticks have been studied in some detail,[20] but its involvement in protein secretion during feeding is unstudied. In other systems, calcium is important to exocytosis.[21] Calreticulins have sequence similarity to a Ca^{2+}-protein that comigrates with an inositol-triphosphate ($InsP_3$)-sensitive Ca^{2+} in HL-60 cells.[22] $InsP_3$ stimulates the release of Ca^{2+} from feeding tick salivary glands.[23] Many secretory cells use $InsP_3$ to generate the Ca^{2+} signal to control either ion permeability or release of granules by exocytosis.[21] A tick calreticulin could play some regulatory role in protein secretion. Calreticulin in tick saliva may be a remnant of protein secretion during feeding.

Tick calreticulin may also exit the cell to enter the saliva by some unconventional secretory mode. Venable et al[24] observed that e-cell granules of the Type III salivary gland acini were not secreted into the lumen of the salivary gland, but were shed into the interstitial spaces, reaching the salivary duct in this manner. In the soft tick, *Argas arboreus*, large granules were released by apocrine secretion.[25] These mechanisms of secretion are unusual, but may result in the secretion of proteins like calreticulin that are found in the endoplasmic reticulum.

Type III acini of the tick salivary glands appear to contain calciosomes (L. Coons, personal communication). Calciosomes have been implicated as storage compartments for Ca^{2+} in the non-muscle cells.[26] The f-cells of the type III salivary acini rapidly enlarge and fill with secretory granules soon after the tick attaches to its host.

Fig. 11.4. (left) Calreticulin homologies (adapted from Michalak et al[19]). A putative nuclear localization site is indicated in italics, residues 187-197; and KPEDWD repeats are indicated in bold, residues 198-203, 215-220, and 232-237. Amino acid sequences for rabbit and human calreticulins are as indicated on the figure. Underlined amino acids in the tick 161A sequence represent differences from rabbit skeletal muscle calreticulin. Clone 161A did not contain 32 amino-terminal residues as shown on figure. RAL-1[38] and Sm-4[39] represent Onchocerca volvulus *and* Schistosoma mansoni *calreticulins, respectively.*

They differentiate into typical glycoprotein secreting cells with extensive endoplasmic reticulum.[27] F-cells actively secrete for two to four days (depending on the tick species), and then undergo autophagy to break down the protein synthesis mechanism. Remarkably, these cells are converted to fluid transport epithelia along with the interstitial cells.[27] Based on the appearance of calreticulin in the salivary glands three days after attachment and the presence of calciosomes, f-cells are a candidate source of this gland protein. Localization studies are in progress to test this hypothesis.

The existence of a secreted calreticulin suggests a novel role for this protein in host-parasite associations. What is calreticulin doing in tick saliva? Arthropod bloodfeeding has been linked to ADP-degrading enzymes like apyrase,[28] which require Ca^{2+} as a cofactor. Elevated Ca^{2+} in the lesion could activate these ADP-degrading enzymes, which could lead to impaired platelet function and augment blood flow into the lesion.[29] This sort of reaction could account for the reactions we observed when ticks were fed on the host immunized with the fusion protein. Calreticulin has antithrombotic activity, which may be actuated by the nitric oxide pathway.[30] Calreticulin as an arthropod secretion could also serve to increase nitric oxide in the feeding lesion, leading to increased vascular permeability. This suggestion seems feasible since Ribeiro et al[31] have demonstrated the presence of nitric oxide in the saliva of the blood sucking bug, *Rhodnius*.

Based on Northern blots and immunoblotting, it appears that at least two isoforms of calreticulin exist in Anopheline mosquitoes and cat fleas (Jaworski et al unpublished data). All arthropods surveyed by immunoblot react with antibody to rabbit skeletal muscle calreticulin. This includes Anopheline mosquitoes (*Anopheles stephensi*), two flea genera (*Ctenocephalides felis* and *Xenopsylla cheopis*), human body louse (*Pediculus humanus*), bedbugs (*Cimex lectularius*), and kissing bugs (*Rhodnius prolixus* and *Triatoma infestans*). Only the salivary glands of mosquitoes, ticks, bedbugs and *X. cheopis* have a crossreactive epitope for the tick-secreted calreticulin (161A). Northern blots of fleas, mosquitoes and *Drosophila* show at least two transcripts for calreticulin at 1.6 and 2.0 kb.

In situ hybridization localizes calreticulin mRNA to the muscle tissue in fleas, mosquitoes and *Drosophila* (Jaworski et al unpublished data). Immunofluorescent antibody assays show a general labeling of insect tissues with calreticulin antibody having several sites of more specific labeling. In fleas, the ovaries are labeled along with the midgut microvilli. The appearance of calreticulin in the ovaries is interesting and remains to be understood. Calreticulin in the flea midgut suggests an alternative source of the protein in flea secretion facilitated by the flea habit of regurgitating into its host during the feeding process. Mosquitoes exhibited highly specific label in the Malpighian tubules. Mosquito Malpighian tubules were also positive with antibody to the tick 161A. All other insect tissues were negative when assayed with anti-161A. The detection of calreticulin in the Malpighian tubules was unexpected. Labeling of Malpighian tubules was not observed in *Drosophila*, a non-blood feeding Dipteran. Salivary gland is the major osmoregulatory organ in ticks, while the Malpighian tubules perform this function for most insects,[32] including adult mosquitoes. As a possible by-product of tick osmoregulation, calreticulin could also work to create the necessary imbalance in host hemostasis for efficient tick feeding. Ixodid ticks take in more than several grams of blood during the early feeding interval—this amount is usually more than 100 times their unfed weight.[12] Securing a blood meal and concentrating this meal by expelling excess water is a challenge for the blood feeding arthropod. It appears calreticulin may play a role in both of these activities. A survey of blood feeding arthropod salivas and in vivo experiments should help to clarify the role of calreticulin in vector arthropods.

Calreticulin in the tick may influence the transmission of pathogens via the blood meal and this possibility is also being studied. We have already shown that calreticulin bound by antibody in the host can dramatically change the feeding site. Such changes are likely to affect pathogen transmission. Saliva-activated transmission (SAT) has been demonstrated in some arthropods (ticks and tick-borne encephalitis virus, TBE;[33] and with sandflies and *Leishmania*, according to Titus and Ribeiro[34]). With TBE, SAT induces changes in the feeding lesion that are used by the virus. SAT was most evident at six days of feeding in an ixodid tick.[35] It is interesting that calreticulin is abundant in the salivary glands at this time.

Finally, calreticulin may be unrecognized by the host as a foreign antigen. Shared antigens exist between endoparasites and hosts.[36,37] However, the possibility of a shared antigen between an arthropod and its vertebrate host has not been investigated. This would be a major adaptation favoring vector success.

REFERENCES

1. Jaworski DC, Simmen FA, Lamoreaux W et al. A secreted calreticulin in ixodid tick saliva. J Insect Physiol 1995; 41:369-375.
2. Jaworski DC, Muller MT, Simmen FA et al. Unfed and early feeding phase salivary gland antigens recognized by antibodies of immune hosts. Exp Parasitol 1990; 70:217-226.
3. Needham GR, Jaworski DC, Sherif N et al. Characterization of ixodid tick salivary gland gene products using recombinant DNA technology. Exp Appl Acarol 1989; 7:21-32.
4. Johnston TH, Bancroft MJ. A tick resistant condition in cattle. Proc R Soc Qd 1918; 30:219-317.
5. Trager W. Further observation on acquired immunity to the tick *Dermacentor variabilis* (Say). J Parasitol 1939; 25:137-139.
6. Fawcett DW, Binnington KC, Voight WP. The cell biology of the ixodid tick salivary gland. In: J.R. Sauer and J.A. Hair, eds. Morphology, Physiology and Behavioral Biology of Ticks, Ellis Horwood, Ltd. Chichester 1986; 22-45.
7. Kaufman WR. Tick-host interaction: a synthesis of current concepts. Parasitology Today 1989; 5:50-59.
8. Jones LD, Hodgson E, Nuttall PA. Enhancement of virus transmission by tick salivary glands. J Gen Virol 1989; 70:1895-1898.
9. Ribeiro JMC. Vector saliva and its role in parasite transmission. Exp Parasitol 1989; 69:104-106.
10. Ribeiro JMC. The role of saliva in tick-host interactions. Exp Applied Acarol 1989; 7:15-20.
11. Ribeiro JMC. Role of saliva in blood-feeding by arthropods. Annu Rev Entomol 1987; 32:463-478.
12. Sonenshine DE. Biology of Ticks, Vol. 1. 1991; p. 155. Oxford Univ. Press, NY.
13. Gordon JR, Allen JR. Factors V and VII anticoagulant activities in the salivary glands of feeding *Dermacentor andersoni* ticks. J Parasitol 1991; 77(1):167-170.
14. Ribeiro JMC, Weis JJ, Telford III, SR. Saliva of the tick *Ixodes dammini* inhibits neutrophil function. Exp Parasitol 1990; 70:382-388.
15. Ribeiro JMC, Makoul GT, Robinson DR. *Ixodes dammini*: evidence for salivary gland prostacyclin. J Parasitol 1988; 74:1068.
16. Ribeiro JMC, Makoul GT, Levine J et al. Antihemostatic, antiinflammatory, and immunosuppressive properties of the salvia of a tick, *Ixodes dammini*. J Exp Med 1985; 161:332-344.
17. Willadsen P, Riding GA. Characterization of a proteolytic-enzyme inhibitor with allergenic activity. Biochem J 1979; 177:41-47.
18. Fliegel L, Burns K, MacLennan DH et al. Molecular cloning of the high-affinity calcium-binding protein (calreticulin) of skeletal muscle sarcoplasmic reticulum. J Biol Chem 1989; 21522-21528.
19. Michalak M, Milner RE, Burns K et al. Calreticulin. Biochem J 1992; 85:681-692.

20. Sauer JR, McSwain JL, Tucker JS et al. Protein phosphorylation and control of tick salivary gland function. Exp Appl Acarol 1989; 7:81-94.

21. Berridge MJ. Inositol triphosphate and diacylglycerol: Two interacting second messengers. Annu Rev Biochem 1987; 56:159-193.

22. Krause KH, Simmerman HKB, Jones LR et al. Sequence similarity of calreticulin with a Ca^{2+}-binding protein that co-purifies with an Ins $(1,4,5)P_3$-sensitive Ca^{2+} store in HL-60 cells. Biochem J 1990; 270:545-548.

23. Roddy CW, McSwain JL, Kocan KM et al. The role of inositol 1, 4, 5-triphosphate in mobilizing intracellular stores in the salivary glands of *Amblyomma americanum* (L.). Insect Biochem 1990; 20:83-89.

24. Venable JH, Webster P, Shapiro SZ et al. An immunocytochemical marker for the complex granules of tick salivary glands which traces e-granule shedding to interstitial labyrinthine spaces. Tiss Cell 1986; 18:765-781.

25. Coons LB, Roshdy MA. Ultrastructure of granule secretion in salivary glands of *Argas (Persicargas) arboreus* during feeding. Z Parasitenkd 1981; 65:225-234.

26. Volpe P, Krause KH, Hashimoto S et al. "Calciosome'" a cytoplasmic organelle: The inositol 1,4,5-triphosphate-sensitive Ca^{2+} store of nonmuscle cells? Proc Natl Acad Sci USA 1988; 85:1091-1095.

27. Fawcett DW, Doxsey SJ, Buscher G. Salivary gland of the tick vector (*Rhipicephalus appendiculatus*) of East Coast fever. I. Ultrastructure of the type III acinus. Tis Cell 1981; 13:209-230.

28. Ribeiro JMC, Rossignol PA, Spielman AJ. Salivary gland apyrase determines probing time in anopheline mosquitoes. J Insect Physiol 1985; 31:689-692.

29. Mustard JF, Packman MA. Normal and abnormal haemostasis. Br Med Bull 1977; 33:187.

30. Benedict C, Kuwahara K, Todd G et al. Calreticulin is a novel antithrombotic agent: blockage of electrically induced coronary thrombosis. Clin Res 1993; 41:275A.

31. Ribeiro JMC, Hazzard JMH, Nussenzveig RH et al. Reversible binding of nitric oxide by a salivary heme protein from a bloodsucking insect. Science 1993; 260:539-541.

32. Chapman RF. The Insects: Structure and Function. 1969, 490-494. American Elsevier , Inc. New York.

33. Jones LD, Kaufman WR, Nuttall PA. Feeding site modification by tick saliva resulting in enhanced virus transmission. Experientia 1992; 48:779-782.

34. Titus RG, Ribeiro JMC. Salivary gland lysates from the sandfly *Lutzomyia longipalpis* enhance *Leishmania* infectivity. Science 1988; 239:1306-1308.

35. Labuda M, Jones LD, Williams T et al. Enhancement of tick-borne encephalitis virus transmission by tick salivary gland extracts. Med Vet Entomol 1993; 7:193-196.

36. Braun G, McKechine MN, Connor V et al. Immunological crossreactivity between a cloned antigen of *Onchocerca volvulus* and a component of the retinal pigment epithelium. J Exp Med 1991; 174:169-177.

37. Clegg JA, Smithers SR, Terry RJ. Acquisitions of human antigens by *Schistosoma mansoni* during cultivation in vitro. Nature 1971; 232:653-654.

38. Unnasch TR, Gallin MY, Soboslay PT et al. Isolation and characterization of expression cDNA clones encoding antigens of *Onchocera volvulus* infective larvae. J Clin Invest 1988; 82:262-269.

39. Khalife J, Trottein F, Schacht A-M et al. Cloning and sequencing of the gene encoding *Schistosoma mansoni* calreticulin. Mol Biochem Parasitol 1993; 57:193-202.

PROTEIN NUCLEAR IMPORT IS MODULATED BY CALRETICULIN

Victor B. Hatcher and Christina Samathanam

PROTEIN NUCLEAR IMPORT

A large number of cellular events occur following the import of proteins into the nucleus from the cytoplasm. Numerous studies have identified protein sequences which act as a signal for protein import into the nucleus.[1-3] Although a specific consensus nuclear signal sequence for protein nuclear import has not been identified, the nuclear localization signal (NLS) usually consists of clusters of arginines, lysines and a helix destabilizing amino acid such as proline or glycine.[4-7] The NLS sequence of SV-40 large T antigen (P-K-K-K-R-K-V) is one example of the prototype of a NLS. The mutation of the second lysine to threonine greatly reduces nuclear import. Some proteins contain split or bipartite NLS with spacer sequences between the NLS sequences. Nucleoplasmin, which contains two clusters of basic amino acids separated by a 10 residue long spacer sequence, is one example of a protein containing a bipartite NLS.[8-10] Some proteins do not contain their own NLS but are shuttled into the nucleus by another protein containing a NLS.[11] Many proteins contain more than one NLS.[12-15] The position of the NLS signal in the protein is important for nuclear import. Protein import does not occur when the NLS is buried in the interior of the protein.[16] Increased protein nuclear import has been observed as the number of NLS sequences increases per protein.[16-20] Modification of the flanking regions near the NLS may modify the rate of protein nuclear import or the total amount of protein imported. Phosphorylation of specific sites can modulate the rate and the amount of protein imported. A casein kinase II phosphorylation site near the SV-40 large T antigen NLS site has been demonstrated to be required to increase the rate of protein nuclear import.[21,22] Phosphorylation of a cdc2 kinase phosphorylation site near the SV-40 large T antigen NLS reduced the total amount of nuclear import.[23] Phosphorylation of dorsal, a Drosophila Rel homolog, may be required for proper nuclear localization of the protein.[24] In addition to a functional NLS, import of protein into the nucleus is dependent on ATP and temperature.[25,26] In the absence of ATP the imported protein binds to the nuclear pore complex but is not imported into the nucleus.[27,28] The binding to the nuclear pore requires a functional NLS. The binding and transport of proteins into the nucleus can be divided into two steps. In the first step, which does not require ATP, the protein containing a NLS binds to the nuclear pore. In the second step, which requires ATP, the imported protein is transported through the nuclear pore into the nucleus. The second step is also temperature dependent.[27,29] Recent studies have demonstrated that the NLS sequence also mediates the outward movement of proteins from the nucleus to the cytoplasm.[30,31]

Protein import into the nucleus can be regulated by masking and unmasking the NLS in proteins. Nuclear import is controlled in the NF-κB family of transcription factors.[32,33] Active NF-κB is present in the nucleus while inactive NF-κB, which binds to the inhibition factor IκB, is found in the cytoplasm. IκB binding to the NLS region masks the NLS in NF-κB, causing the NF-κB to be retained in the cytoplasm. Phosphorylation disrupts the IκB-NF-κB complex, exposing the NLS in the NF-κB, and NF-κB enters the nucleus.[33] In several proteins one part of the molecule causes the protein domain containing the NLS to be inaccessible.[34-37] NF-κB is one example. NF-κB is a dimer containing subunits p50 and p65 in which p50 has a precursor, p110. In the precursor p110 the NLS is inaccessible and p110 resides in the cytoplasm. When the p110 is cleaved exposing the NLS, nuclear localization occurs.[38-41] The glucocorticoid receptor, a zinc finger type DNA-binding protein which regulates transcription, is another example of a protein in which nuclear protein import is regulated. In the absence of hormone the receptor which contains NLS and a second signal domain resides in the cytoplasm.[42,43] In the presence of hormone the NLS become active and the glucocorticoid receptor moves into the nucleus. The NLS becomes accessible and active in the presence of hormones in the human androgen receptor,[43-45] in the rabbit progesterone receptor[46] but not in the estrogen receptor.[47] Two cytosolic polypeptides (60-kDa, 70-kDa) that bind to the glucocorticoid or thyroid hormone receptor NLS have been identified.[48] Heat shock proteins have been implicated in protein nuclear import. Heat shock cognate protein 70 (hscp70) and heat shock protein 70 (hsp70), which can bind to NLS peptides, have been implicated in nuclear import.[49-51] Proteins related to hsp70 shuttle between the nucleus and the cytoplasm of *Xenopus* oocytes.[52,53] Hsp70 which binds to the oncoprotein, myc; when coexpressed they accumulate in the nucleus.[54,55] Heat shock can cause the glucocorticoid receptor to move to the nucleus in the absence of hormone.[56]

The presence of an NLS sequence in the protein suggests that a NLS-recognition factor must exist either at the nuclear pore or in the cytosolic fraction. An NLS recognition factor in the cytoplasm could shuttle the protein to the nuclear pore. Several proteins that interact with NLS peptides and promote protein nuclear import in several models of nuclear import have been identified.[57] Two cytosolic proteins (60-kDa, 70-kDa) have been identified which bind to the SV-40 T large antigen NLS sequence.[58] Two cytosolic proteins which promote nuclear import in permeabilized cells were NEM-sensitive while a third cytosolic factor was NEM-insensitive. A NLS-binding phosphoprotein (70-kDa) was required for nuclear import in permeabilized Drosophila cells.[59] A human cytoplasm NLS binding protein (70-kDa) has also been identified.[60] Several NLS binding proteins have been localized in the nucleus and may function in targeting proteins to the nucleus.[61-63] Cytoplasmic factors are required for binding to the nuclear pore.[64,65] The product of the yeast gene NIP1 is found in the cytoplasm and is required for nuclear import.[66] Two NEM-sensitive factors, NIF-1 and NIF-2 are required for nuclear import. NIF-1 is required for nuclear pore binding and works with NIF-2 to promote nuclear import. One of the cytosolic factors required for nuclear import interacts with two different O-glycosylated nucleoporins. The nucleoporins are the proteins which reside in the nuclear pore. One cytosolic factor binds to one of the proteins, Nup153 (p180), found on the intranuclear side of the nuclear pore.[67] Ran/TC4, a member of the Ras family of small GTP-binding proteins which is localized in the nucleus and cytoplasm, has been identified as one of the soluble factors required for nuclear import.[68,69] It has been observed that the microinjection of purified SV40 large T antigen into the cytoplasm of BALB/c 3T3 cells significantly increased both the rate of signal-mediated nuclear transport and the functional size of the transport channels that are located within the pores.[70] Mutants of SV40 large T antigen which were unable to promote the increase in nuclear transport were unable to bind p53. The studies suggested that p53, a protien associated with tumor suppression, might act as a nuclear transport suppressor. Several other cytosolic factors have been identified which promote protein nuclear import.[71,72] The function that the different cytosolic factors play in nuclear pore binding and translocation into the nucleus is not clear.

The nuclear pores which are involved in protein nuclear import and connect the nucleus to the cytoplasm have been extensively investigated, with emphasis on structure and function.[73-77] The nuclear pore has been divided into four separate structural elements. Short thick filaments are attached to the cytoplasmic side of the pore and may be involved in the initial docking process. The scaffold includes the majority of the pore. The scaffold maintains the fusion of the two nuclear membranes and creates the 900 Å hole in the nuclear envelope. In addition, the scaffold provides the 90 Å diffusional channel and supports the smaller central transporter that regulates import and export. The central plug or transporter carries out the function of active transport of the proteins. The central plug or transporter is observed as a proteinaceous ring which can be resolved into several distinct conformations. It has been suggested that a protein binds to the periphery of the transporter ring, moves and docks in the central channel, which causes the channel to open, and translocates through the open channel. The transporter, which consists of two irises of eight arms each stacked on top of each other, could act like a diaphragm of a camera. The imported protein would dock on the short thick filaments on the nuclear pore, a signal would open the first iris, the protein would move into the pore, the second iris would open and the protein would move further, the first iris would close and the protein would move into the nucleus. A basket is attached to the nucleoplasmic side of the pore, but the function of the basket with respect to protein transport is not clear. Studies have been performed on the proteins of the nuclear pore complex, the nucleoporins. A large number of nucleoporins contain O-linked N-acetylglucosamine residues which can interact with the lectin wheat germ agglutinin. Inhibition of in vitro nuclear protein import has been observed with wheat germ agglutinin.[78] One of the glycoproteins gp210, an integral membrane protein, is thought to attach the nuclear pore complex to the nuclear membrane.[79-81] When antibodies were produced to the lumenal domain of gp210, protein nuclear transport and diffusion were inhibited.[82] A monoclonal antibody against a novel class of nuclear pore proteins also inhibited nuclear import.[83] Several nucleoporins have been identified, including p62 and Nup153 in vertebrates.[84-87] Nucleoporin genes cloned from yeast may represent new families of nucleoporins.[88-90] Although numerous nucleoporins have been identified and characterized, the majority of the nucleoporins in the nuclear pore complex have not been investigated.

CALRETICULIN AND PROTEIN NUCLEAR IMPORT

Calreticulin, a Ca^{2+}-binding multifunctional protein, has been localized in the lumen of the endoplasmic reticulin and in the nucleus.[91,92] The normal cellular function of calreticulin has not been elucidated. Calreticulin and calreticulin-like molecules have been implicated in a variety of cellular functions. Calreticulin has been identified as one of the proteins which respond to heat shock.[93] Heat shock, induced glycosylation of calreticulin has been demonstrated.[94,95] Calreticulin has also been induced in renal epithelial cells by amino acid deprivation.[96] Calreticulin, which has been detected on the surface of neutrophils, decreases during neutrophil stimulation, probably due to shedding of the calreticulin.[97] Infection of fibroblasts with cytomyolovirus increased cell surface expression of calreticulin.[98] During rubella virus RNA replication a homologue of calreticulin was identified as one of the binding proteins which interact with *cis*-acting elements of the virus (Chapter 7).[99] Thus, calreticulin is one of the response elements to stress in a large number of cells. Studies have demonstrated that calreticulin is an autoantigen (Chapter 8),[100-102] and patients with systemic lupus erythematosus (SLE) produce antibodies to calreticulin. Currently it is controversial whether calreticulin is one of the Ro-SS/A autoantigens present in patients with SLE and Sjögren's Syndrome.[103-105] Calreticulin can interact with the α-subunit of integrin receptors via the highly conserved K-L-G-F-F-K-R sequence in the cytoplasmic domain.[106,107] These studies suggest a fundamental role of calreticulin in cell-intracellular matrix interactions.[108] Calreticulin involvement has been implicated with specific functions of lymphocytes (Chapter 9).[109] Cytolytic T lymphocytes are cytolytic cells known to release the cytolytic protein perforin and the granzyme proteases, following interaction with target cells. Calreticulin is a constituent of the lytic granules in cytolytic T lymphocytes and may prevent autolysis. Activation of T-lymphocytes correlates with increased expression of calreticulin[110-112] and with structural and functional changes in intracellular Ca^{2+} stores. In the neuroblastoma X glioma NG-108-15 whose cells calreticulin expression was decreased with antisense oligonucleotides had lowered Ca^{2+} response to bradykinin and increased sensitivity to ionomycin. The study demonstrated that the level of calreticulin expression was directly related to the Ca^{2+} storage capacity of the inositol 1,4,5-trisphosphate-sensitive Ca^{2+} pool. A relationship may exist between the level of calreticulin and the protection against cytotoxic calcium overload. Recent studies have suggested that calreticulin may function in regulating gene expression (Chapter 6). The N-terminus of calreticulin interacts with the DNA-binding domain of the glucocorticoid receptor and prevents the receptor from binding to the glucocorticoid expression element.[113] Overexpression of calreticulin in mouse L fibroblasts inhibits glucocorticoid-response-mediated transcriptional activation of a glucocorticoid-sensitive reporter gene and of the endogenous glucocorticoid-sensitive gene encoding cytochrome P450. It has also been demonstrated that calreticulin inhibits the binding of the androgen receptor to its hormone-responsive DNA element.[114] Calreticulin inhibits androgen receptor and retinoic acid receptor transcriptional activities in vivo as well as retinoic acid-induced neuronal differentiation.

We have been investigating factors involved in modulating protein nuclear transport in human umbilical vein endothelial cells (HUVEC) and in NRK (normal rat kidney) cells. A nuclear import model was set up in HUVEC and NRK cells using either the fluorescent phycobiliprotein allophycocyanin (APC) conjugated to synthetic peptides containing a NLS sequence, rhodamine labeled acidic fibroblast growth factor (R-FGF-1), or rhodamine labeled recombinant calreticulin.[71,72] Peptides were synthesized containing the NLS from SV-40 large T antigen (CGGGPKKKRKVED), the NLS from FGF-1 (CGGGNYKKPKL) and the mutant transport-deficient NLS from SV-40 large T antigen (CGGGPK<u>N</u>KRKVED). Each peptide was linked separately to the APC molecule so that there were between 10-15 peptides per APC molecule. The model was set up using digitonin (40 μg/ml) permeabilized NRK cells, digitonin (40 μg/ml) permeabilized HUVEC and reticulocyte lysate as the source of cytosol. The complete transport mixture contained untreated reticulocyte lysate dialyzed and diluted to give the following final conditions: 25-35 mg/ml protein, 50 μg APC-peptide conjugate, 20 mM Hepes, pH 7.3, 110 mM potassium acetate, 5 mM sodium acetate, 2 mM DTT, 1 mM EGTA, 1 mM ATP, 5 mM creatine phosphate, 20 U/ml creatine phosphokinase, 1 μg/ml each aprotinin, leupeptin and pepstatin in a total volume of 500 μl. The incubation of complete transport mixture with the cells was performed at 30°C for 30 min with 60 μl of complete transport mixture and 6 μg APC conjugate. Normaski differential

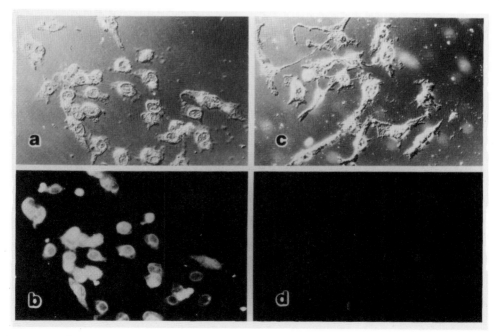

Fig. 12. 1. Nuclear import in HUVEC: (a) (b) Complete transport mixture with APC-CGGGPKKKRKVED; (c) (d) Complete transport mixture with APC-CGGGPK<u>N</u>KRVED: (a) (c) Normaski DIC optics; (b) (d) Fluorescence microscopy.

interference contrast (DIC) optics or phase contrast microscopy and fluorescence microscopy of the treated cells was performed utilizing a Zeiss Axioplat microscope in the Ultrastructural Core Facility. Significant amounts of nuclear import were observed in HUVEC with APC-CGGGPKKKRKVED, while no import was observed with APC-CGGGPKNKRKVED (Fig. 12.1). In our experiments, the uptake was temperature dependent in that no import was observed at 4°C (Fig. 12.2). No nuclear import was observed when ATP was removed from the reaction mixture (Fig. 12.2). Nuclear import was also performed utilizing either 3 µg, 6 µg or 9 µg of APC-CGGGPKKKRKVED in NRK cells (Fig. 12.3). Increased nuclear import was observed with increased APC-peptide concentrations. We have also investigated the import of the synthesized peptide containing the FGF-1 nuclear location signal (CGGGNYKKPKL) linked to APC. The uptake of APC-CGGGNYKKPKL was temperature and ATP dependent in NRK cells and HUVEC cells.

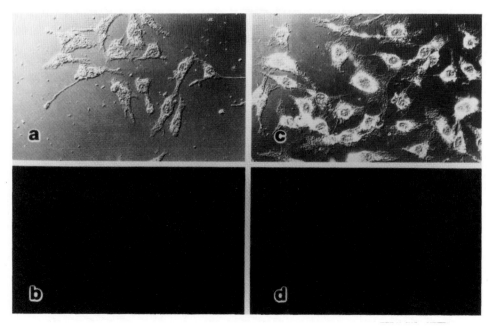

Fig. 12.2. Nuclear import in HUVEC: (a) (b) Complete transport mixture with APC-CGGGPKKKRKVED at 4 °C; (c) (d) Complete transport mixture with APC-CGGGPKKKRKVED minus ATP,m at 30 °C: (a) (c) Normaski DIC optics; (b) (d) Fluorescence microscopy.

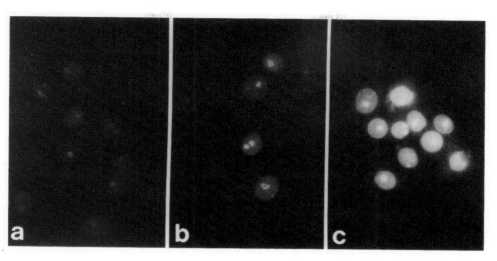

Fig. 12.3. Nuclear import of APC-CGGGPKKKRKVED in NRK cells: Complete transport mixture with either (a) 3 µg APC-peptide (b) 6 µg APC-peptide or (c) 9 µg APC-peptide. Fluorescence microscopy.

The import model was utilized to investigate the role of calreticulin in nuclear import. Calreticulin (1 µg/µl) was added to the transport mixture (500 µl) and an aliquot (60 µl) tested on the import of APC-CGGGNYKKPKL in digitonin treated HUVEC and import of APC-CGGGNYKKPKL in digitonin-treated NRK cells. Calreticulin (120 ng) promoted the import of the peptides containing the FGF-1 nuclear localization signal conjugated to APC (APC-CGGGNYKKPKL) in HUVEC and NRK cells. Identical experimental conditions were used in the cells in which calreticulin was added to the transport mixture. In the import studies, conditions were chosen so that maximal import of APC-conjugated peptides was not observed in the absence of calreticulin. The effect of calreticulin on nuclear import of APC-CGGGNYKKPKL in HUVEC is shown in Figure 12.4. In Figure 12.4A,C phase contrast microscopy of digitonin-treated HUVEC cells is illustrated. No morphological differences were observed between non-treated and calreticulin (120 ng/60 µl) treated cells. A significant increase in the nuclear fluorescence was observed in the HUVEC cells in which the transport mixture contained calreticulin (Fig. 12.4D). The results suggest that during the 30 min incubation period a significant increase in the nuclear import of APC conjugated to a peptide containing the NLS was observed in the presence of calreticulin. Similar results were observed with NRK cells (Fig. 12.5)

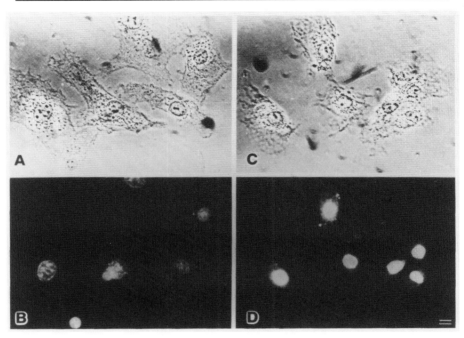

Fig. 12.4. Stimulation of the nuclear accumulation of APC-CGGGNYKKPKL by purified calreticulin in HUVEC: (A) (B) Complete transport mixture with APC-CGGGNYKKPKL; (C) (D) plus calreticulin (120 ng) added to the reaction mixture (60 µl): (A) (C) Phase contrast microscopy; (B) (D) Fluorescence microscopy.

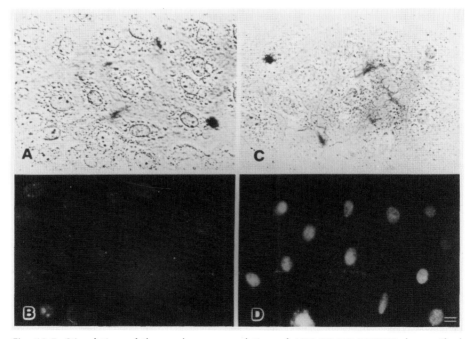

Fig. 12.5. Stimulation of the nuclear accumulation of APC-CGGGNYKKPKL by purified calreticulin in NRK cells: (A) (B) Complete transport mixture with APC-CGGGNYKKPKL; (C) (D) plus calreticulin (120 ng) added to the reaction mixture (60 µl): (A) (C) Phase contrast microscopy; (B) (D) Fluorescence microscopy.

and with peptides containing the SV-40 T large antigen NLS conjugated to APC in HUVEC and NRK cells (results not shown). Calreticulin promoted the nuclear import of APC conjugated to nuclear localization signals in digitonin-treated NRK cells and HUVEC. The studies have been repeated with rhodamine labeled acidic fibroblast growth factor (10 μg) (R-FGF-1). The uptake was temperature and ATP dependent in HUVEC. In HUVEC, R-FGF-1 also localized in the cytoplasm. Again, calreticulin promoted the nuclear uptake of R-FGF-1 in HUVEC (Fig. 12.6). We investigated whether calreticulin alone would be imported into the nucleus in permeabilized HUVEC since calreticulin contains a NLS sequence.[91] The results demonstrated that under identical conditions rhodamine labeled recombinant calreticulin (10 μg) was imported into the nucleus (Fig. 12.7). Calreticulin is imported into the nucleus when calreticulin is added to the import mixture containing reticulocyte lysate and ATP.

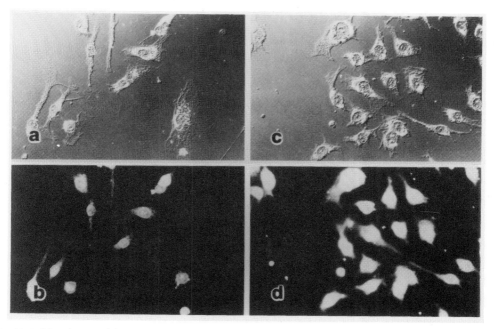

Fig. 12.6. Stimulation of the nuclear accumulation of rhodamine labeled acidic fibroblast growth factor (R-FGF-1) by purified calreticulin in HUVEC: (a) (b) Complete transport mixture minus the APC conjugate plus R-FGF-1 (10 μg); (c) (d) plus calreticulin (120 ng) added to the reaction mixture (60μl): (a) (c) Normaski DIC optics; (b) (d) Fluorescence microscopy.

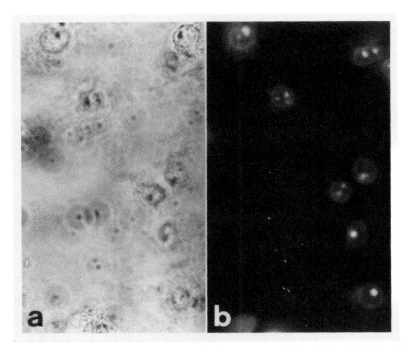

Fig. 12.7. Nuclear import of rhodamine labeled calreticulin (R-CRT) in HUVEC with complete transport mixture minus the APC-conjugate plus R-CRT: (a) Phase contrast microscopy; (b) Fluorescence microscopy.

The molecular mechanism by which calreticulin promotes protein nuclear import is not understood. Calreticulin could interact with the NLS of the imported protein in the cytoplasm or at the nuclear pore and shuttle the protein into the nucleus. Calreticulin could also interact with a natural inhibitor of nuclear transport, resulting in significant increase in nuclear transport.

ACKNOWLEDGMENTS

Supported by Grants-in-Aid from The American Heart Association, National Center and American Heart Association, New York City Affiliate, a research grant from The Arthritis Foundation and NIH grants HL37025 and HL02990. Recombinant calreticulin was supplied by Marek Michalak, University of Alberta, Edmonton, Alberta. We thank Jayesh Shah for technical support and Eileen Rubinstein for thoughtful suggestions and secretarial assistance.

REFERENCES

1. DeRobertis EM, Longthorne RF, Gurdon JB. Intracellular migration of nuclear proteins in *Xenopus oocytes*. Nature 1978; 272:254-256.
2. Garcia-Bustos J, Heitman J, Hall MN. Nuclear protein localization. Biochim Biophys Acta 1991; 1071:83-101.
3. Silver PA. How proteins enter the nucleus. Cell 1991; 64:489-497.
4. Lanford RE, Butel JS. Construction and characterization of an SV40 mutant defective in nuclear transport of T antigen. Cell 1984; 37:801-813.
5. Kalderon D, Richardson WD, Markham AF et al. Sequence requirements for nuclear location of simian virus 40 large T-antigen. Nature 1984; 311:33-38.
6. Kalderon D, Roberts BL, Richardson WD et al. A short amino acid sequence able to specify nuclear location. Cell 1984; 39:499-509.
7. Chelsky D, Ralph R, Jonak G. Sequence requirements for synthetic peptide-mediated translocation to the nucleus. Mol Cell Biol 1989; 9:2487-2489.
8. Dingwall C, Robbins J, Dilworth SM et al. The nucleoplasmin nuclear location sequence is larger and more complex than that of SV40 large T-antigen. J Cell Biol 1988; 107:841-849.
9. Robbins J, Dilworth SM, Lasky RA et al. Two independent basic domains in nucleoplasmin nuclear targeting sequence: Identification of a class of bipartite nuclear targeting sequences. Cell 1991; 64:615-623.
10. Dingwall C, Lasky RA. Nuclear targeting sequences - a consensus. TIBS 1991; 16:478-481.
11. Zhao L, Padmanabhan R. Nuclear transport of adenovirus DNA polymerase is facilitated by interaction with preterminal protein. Cell 1988; 55:1005-1015.
12. Richardson WD, Roberts BL, Smith AE. Nuclear location signals in polyoma virus large T-cell. Cell 1986; 44:77-85.
13. Dang CV, Lee WMF. Identification of the human c-myc protein nuclear translocation signal. Mol Cell Biol 1988; 8:4048-4054.
14. Morin N, Delsert C, Klessig DF. Nuclear localization in the adenovirus DNA binding protein: Requirement for two signals and complementation during viral infection. Mol Cell Biol 1989; 9:4372-4380.
15. Underwood MR, Fried HM. Characterization of nuclear localizing sequences derived from yeast ribosomol protein L29. EMBO J 1990; 9:91-99.
16. Roberts BL, Richardson WD, Smith AE. The effect of protein content on nuclear location signal function. Cell 1987; 58:466-475.

17. Lanford RE, Kanda P, Kennedy RC. Induction of nuclear transport with a synthetic peptide homologous to the SV 40 T-antigen transport signal. Cell 1986; 46:575-582.

18. Dworetzky SI, Lanford RE, Feldherr CM. The effects of variations in the number and sequence of targeting signals in nuclear uptake. J Cell Biol 1988; 107:1279-1287.

19. Finlay DR, Newmeyer DD, Hartl PM et al. Nuclear transportation in vitro. J Cell Sci 1989; 11:225-242.

20. Lanford RE, Feldherr CM, White RG et al. Comparison of diverse transport signals in synthetic-induced nuclear transport. Exp Cell Res 1990; 186:32-38.

21. Rihs HP, Peters R. Nuclear transport kinetics depend on phosphorylation site-containing sequences flanking the karyophilic signal of the simian virus 40 T-antigen. EMBO J 1989; 8:1479-1489.

22. Rihs HP, Jans DA, Fan H et al. The rate of nuclear cytoplasmic protein transport is determined by the casein kinase II site flanking the nuclear localization sequence of the SV 40 T-antigen. EMBO J 1991; 10:633-639.

23. Jans DA, Ackermann MJ, Bischoff JR et al. p34 cdc2-mediated phosphorylation at T 124 inhibits nuclear import of SV 40 T-antigen proteins. J Cell Biol 1991; 115:1203-1212.

24. Gillespie SK, Wasserman SA. Dorsal, a Drosophila Rel-like protein, is phosphorylated upon activation of the transmembrane protein Toll. Mol Cell Biol 1994; 14:3559-3568.

25. Newmeyer DD, Finlay DR, Forbes DJ. In vitro transport of a fluorescent nuclear protein and exclusion of non-nuclear proteins. J Cell Biol 1986; 103:2091-2092.

26. Newmeyer DD, Lucocq JM, Burglin TR et al. Assembly in vitro of nuclei active in nuclear protein transport: ATP is required for nucleoplasmin accumulation. EMBO J 1986; 5:501-510.

27. Newmeyer DD, Forbes DJ. Nuclear import can be separated into distinct steps in vivo: Nuclear pore binding and translocation. Cell 1988; 52:641-653.

28. Richardson WD, Mills AD, Dilworth SM et al. Nuclear protein migration involves two steps: Rapid binding at the nuclear envelope followed by slower translocation through nuclear pores. Cell 1988; 88:655-664.

29. Breeuwer M, Goldfarb DS. Facilitated nuclear transport of histone H1 and other small nucleophilic proteins. Cell 1990; 60:999-1000.

30. Guiochon-Mantel A, Delabre K, Lescop P et al. Nuclear localization signals also mediate the outward movement of proteins from the nucleus. Proc Natl Acad Sci USA 1994; 91:7179-7183.

31. Madan AP, DeFranco DB. Bidirectional transport of glucocorticoid receptors across the nuclear envelope. Proc Natl Acad Sci USA 1993; 90:3588-3592.

QUESTIONNAIRE

Receive a FREE BOOK of your choice

Please help us out—Just answer the questions below, then select the book of your choice from the list on the back and return this card.

R.G. Landes Company publishes five book series: *Medical Intelligence Unit, Molecular Biology Intelligence Unit, Neuroscience Intelligence Unit, Tissue Engineering Intelligence Unit* and *Biotechnology Intelligence Unit.* We also publish comprehensive, shorter than book-length reports on well-circumscribed topics in molecular biology and medicine. The authors of our books and reports are acknowledged leaders in their fields and the topics are unique. Almost without exception, there are no other comprehensive publications on these topics.

Our goal is to publish material in important and rapidly changing areas of bioscience for sophisticated scientists. To achieve this goal, we have accelerated our publishing program to conform to the fast pace in which information grows in bioscience. Most of our books and reports are published within 90 to 120 days of receipt of the manuscript.

Please circle your response to the questions below.

1. We would like to sell our *books* to scientists and students at a deep discount. But we can only do this as part of a prepaid subscription program. The retail price range for our books is $59-$99. Would you pay $196 to select four *books* per year from any of our Intelligence Units–$49 per book–as part of a prepaid program?

    Yes   No

2. We would like to sell our *reports* to scientists and students at a deep discount. But we can only do this as part of a prepaid subscription program. The retail price range for our reports is $39-$59. Would you pay $145 to select five *reports* per year–$29 per report–as part of a prepaid program?

    Yes   No

3. Would you pay $39–the retail price range of our books is $59-$99–to receive any single book in our Intelligence Units if it is spiral bound, but in every other way identical to the more expensive hardcover version?

    Yes   No

To receive your free book, please fill out the shipping information below, select your free book choice from the list on the back of this survey and mail this card to:

R.G. Landes Company, 909 S. Pine Street, Georgetown, Texas 78626 U.S.A.

Your Name _____

Address _____

City_____ State/Province:_____

Country: _____ Postal Code:_____

My computer type is Macintosh_____ ; IBM-compatible _____ ; Other _____

Do you own ____ or plan to purchase ___ a CD-ROM drive?

Available Free Titles

Please check three titles in order of preference.
Your request will be filled based on availability. Thank you.

☐ Water Channels
Alan Verkman,
University of California-San Francisco

☐ The Na,K-ATPase:
Structure-Function Relationship
J.-D. Horisberger, University of Lausanne

☐ Intrathymic Development of T Cells
J. Nikolic-Zugic,
Memorial Sloan-Kettering Cancer Center

☐ Cyclic GMP
Thomas Lincoln, University of Alabama

☐ Primordial VRM System and the Evolution
of Vertebrate Immunity
John Stewart, Institut Pasteur-Paris

☐ Thyroid Hormone Regulation
of Gene Expression
Graham R. Williams, University of Birmingham

☐ Mechanisms of Immunological Self Tolerance
Guido Kroemer, CNRS Génétique Moléculaire et
Biologie du Développement-Villejuif

☐ The Costimulatory Pathway
for T Cell Responses
Yang Liu, New York University

☐ Molecular Genetics of Drosophila Oogenesis
Paul F. Lasko, McGill University

☐ Mechanism of Steroid Hormone Regulation
of Gene Transcription
M.-J. Tsai & Bert W. O'Malley, Baylor University

☐ Liver Gene Expression
François Tronche & Moshe Yaniv,
Institut Pasteur-Paris

☐ RNA Polymerase III Transcription
R.J. White, University of Cambridge

☐ src Family of Tyrosine Kinases in Leukocytes
Tomas Mustelin, La Jolla Institute

☐ MHC Antigens and NK Cells
Rafael Solana & Jose Peña,
University of Córdoba

☐ Kinetic Modeling of Gene Expression
James L. Hargrove, University of Georgia

☐ PCR and the Analysis of the T Cell Receptor
Repertoire
Jorge Oksenberg, Michael Panzara & Lawrence
Steinman, Stanford University

☐ Myointimal Hyperplasia
Philip Dobrin, Loyola University

☐ Transgenic Mice as an In Vivo Model
of Self-Reactivity
David Ferrick & Lisa DiMolfetto-Landon,
University of California-Davis and Pamela Ohashi,
Ontario Cancer Institute

☐ Cytogenetics of Bone and Soft Tissue Tumors
Avery A. Sandberg, Genetrix & Julia A. Bridge ,
University of Nebraska

☐ The Th1-Th2 Paradigm and Transplantation
Robin Lowry, Emory University

☐ Phagocyte Production and Function Following
Thermal Injury
Verlyn Peterson & Daniel R. Ambruso,
University of Colorado

☐ Human T Lymphocyte Activation Deficiencies
José Regueiro, Carlos Rodríguez-Gallego
and Antonio Arnaiz-Villena,
Hospital 12 de Octubre-Madrid

☐ Monoclonal Antibody in Detection and
Treatment of Colon Cancer
Edward W. Martin, Jr., Ohio State University

☐ Enteric Physiology of the Transplanted Intestine
Michael Sarr & Nadey S. Hakim, Mayo Clinic

☐ Artificial Chordae in Mitral Valve Surgery
Claudio Zussa, S. Maria dei Battuti Hospital-Treviso

☐ Injury and Tumor Implantation
Satya Murthy & Edward Scanlon,
Northwestern University

☐ Support of the Acutely Failing Liver
A.A. Demetriou, Cedars-Sinai

☐ Reactive Metabolites of Oxygen and Nitrogen
in Biology and Medicine
Matthew Grisham, Louisiana State-Shreveport

☐ Biology of Lung Cancer
Adi Gazdar & Paul Carbone,
Southwestern Medical Center

☐ Quantitative Measurement
of Venous Incompetence
Paul S. van Bemmelen, Southern Illinois University
and John J. Bergan, Scripps Memorial Hospital

☐ Adhesion Molecules in Organ Transplants
Gustav Steinhoff, University of Kiel

☐ Purging in Bone Marrow Transplantation
Subhash C. Gulati,
Memorial Sloan-Kettering Cancer Center

☐ Trauma 2000: Strategies for the New Millennium
David J. Dries & Richard L. Gamelli,
Loyola University

32. Baeuerle PA, Baltimore D. Activation of DNA-binding activity in an apparently cytoplasmic precursor of the NF-κB transcription factor. Cell 1988; 53:211-217.
33. Ghosh S, Baltimore D. Activation in vitro of NF-κB by phosphorylation of its inhibitor IκB. Nature 1990; 344:678-682.
34. Eldar H, BenChaim J, Liunch E. Deletions in the regulatory or kinase domains of protein kinase C-alpha cause association with the cell nucleus. Exp Cell Res 1992; 202:259-266.
35. Roberts BL, Richardson WD, Smith AE. The effect of context on nuclear location signal function. Cell 1987; 50:465-475.
36. Restrepo-Hartwig MA, Carrington JC. Regulation of nuclear transport of a plant potyvirus protein by auto proteolysis. J Virol 1992; 66:5662-5666.
37. Gao M, Knipe DM. Distal protein sequences can affect the function of a nuclear localization signal. Mol Cell Biol 1992; 12:1330-1339.
38. Naumann M, Wulczyn FG, Scheidereit C. The NF-κB precursor p105 and the proto-oncogene product Bcl-2 are IκB molecules and control nuclear translocation of NF-κB. EMBO J 1993; 12:213-222.
39. Beg AA, Ruben SM, Scheinman RI et al. IκB interacts with the nuclear localization sequences of the subunits of NF-κB, a mechanism for cytoplasmic retention. Genes Dev 1992; 6:1899-1913.
40. Zabel U, Henkel T, Dos Santos SM et al. Nuclear uptake control of NF-κB by MAD-3 and IκB protein present in the nucleus. EMBO J 1993; 12:201-211.
41. Ganchi PA, Sun SC, Greene WC et al. IκB/MAD-3 masks the nuclear localization signal of NF-κB, p65 and requires the transactivation domain to inhibit NF-κB p65 DNA binding. Mol Biol Cell 1992; 3:1339-1352.
42. Picard D, Yamamoto KR. Two signals mediate hormone-dependent nuclear localization of the glucocorticoid receptor. EMBO J 1987; 6:3333-3760.
43. Picard D, Kumart V, Chambont P et al. Signal transduction by steroid hormones: Nuclear localization is differentially regulated in estrogen and glucocortoid receptors. Cell Reg 1990; 1:291-299.
44. Jenster G, Trapman J, Brinkman AO. Nuclear import of the human androgen receptor. Biochem J 1993; 293:761-768.
45. Zhou ZX, Sar M, Simental JA et al. A ligand-dependent bipartite nuclear targeting signal in the human androgen receptor. Requirement for the DNA-binding domain and modulation by NH_2-terminal and carboxyl-terminal sequences. J Biol Chem 1994; 269:13115-13123.
46. Guiochon-Mantel A, Zoosfelt H, Lescop P et al. Mechanisms of nuclear localization of the progesterone receptor. Evidence for interaction between monomers. Cell 1989; 57:1147-1154.

47. Simental JA, Sar M, Lane MV et al. Transcriptional activation and nuclear targeting signals of the hormone estrogen receptor. J Biol Chem 1991; 266:510-518.

48. LaCasse EC, Lochnan HA, Walker P et al. Identification of binding proteins for nuclear localization signals of the glucocorticoid and thyroid hormone receptors. Endocrinology 1993; 132:1017-1025.

49. Shi Y, Thomas JO. The transport of proteins into the nucleus requires the 70-kilo dalton heat shock protein or its cytosolic cognate. Mol Cell Biol 1992; 12:2186-2192.

50. Imamoto-Sonobe N, Matsuoka Y, Semba T et al. A protein recognized by antibodies to Asp-Asp-Asp-Glu-Asp shows specific binding activity to heterogeneous nuclear transport signals. J Biol Chem 1990; 265:16504-16508.

51. Imamoto N, Matsuoka Y, Kurihara T at al. Antibodies against 70-kD heat shock cognate protein inhibit mediated nuclear transport of karyophilic proteins. J Cell Biol 1992; 119:1047-1061.

52. Mandell RB, Feldherr CM. Identification of two hsp-70 related Xenopus oocyte proteins that are capable of recycling across the nuclear envelope. J Cell Biol 1990; 111:1775-1783.

53. Mandell RB, Feldherr CM. The effect of carboxyl-terminal deletions on the nuclear transport of rat hsp70. Exp Cell Res 1992; 198:164-169.

54. Henriksson M, Classon M, Axelson H et al. Nuclear colocalization of c-myc protein and hsp70 in cells transfected with human wild-type and mutant c-myc genes. Exp Cell Res 1992; 203:383-394.

55. Koskinen PJ, Sistonen I, Evan G et al. Nuclear colocalization of cellular and viral myc proteins with hsp70 in myc-overexpressing cells. J Virol 1991; 65:842-851.

56. Sanchez ER. Heat shock induces translocation to the nucleus of the unliganded glucocorticoid receptor. J Biol Chem 1992; 267:17-20.

57. Yamasaki L, Lanford RE. Nuclear transport: a guide in import receptors. TICB 1992; 2:123-127.

58. Adam SA, Gerace L. Cytosolic proteins that specifically bind nuclear location signals are receptors for nuclear import. Cell 1991; 66:837-847.

59. Stochaj U, Silver PA. A conserved phosphoprotein that specifically binds nuclear localization sequences is involved in nuclear import. J Cell Biol 1992; 117:473-482.

60. Li R, Shi Y, Thomas JO. Intracellular distribution of a nuclear localization binding protein. Exp Cell Res 1992; 202:355-365.

61. Lee WC, Melese T. Identification and characterization of a nuclear localization sequence binding protein in yeast. Proc Natl Acad Sci USA 1989; 86:8808-8812.

62. Lee WC, Xue ZX, Melese T. The NSR1 gene encodes a protein that specifically binds nuclear localization sequences and has two RNA recognition motifs. J Cell Biol 1991; 113:1-12.

63. Meier UT, Blobel G. A nuclear localization signal binding protein in the nucleolus. J Cell Biol 1990; 111:2235-2245.

64. Moore MS, Blobel G. The two steps of nuclear import, targeting to the nuclear envelope and translocation through the nuclear pore, require different cytosolic factors. Cell 1992; 69:939-950.

65. Akey CW, Goldfarb DS. Protein import through the nuclear pore complex is a multistep process. J Cell Biol 1989; 109:971-982.

66. Gu Z, Moerschell RP, Sherman F et al. NIP1 gene required for nuclear transport in yeast. Proc Natl Acad Sci USA 1992; 89:10355-10359.

67. Sterne-Marr R, Blevitt JM, Gerace L. O-linked glycoproteins of the nuclear pore complex interact with a cytosolic factor required for nuclear protein import. J Cell Biol 1992; 116:271-280.

68. Melchior F, Paschal B, Evan J et al. Inhibition of nuclear protein import by nonhydrolyzable analogues of GTP and identification of the small GTPase Ran/TC4 as an essential transport factor. J Cell Biol 1993; 123:1649-1659.

69. Moore MS, Blobel G. A G protein involved in nucleocytoplasmic transport: the role of Ran. Trends Biochem Sci 1994; 19:211-216.

70. Feldherr C, Cole C, Lanford RE et al. The effects of SV40 large T antigen and p53 on nuclear transport capacity in BALB/c 3T3 cells. Exp Cell Res 1994; 213:164-171.

71. Adam SA, Sterne-Marr R, Gerace L. Nuclear protein import in permeabilized mammalian cells requires soluble cytoplasmic factors. J Cell Biol 1990; 111:807-816.

72. Adam SA, Sterne-Marr R, Gerace L. In vitro nuclear protein import using permeabilized mammalian cells. Meth Cell Biol 1991; 35:469-482.

73. Forbes DJ. Structure and function of the nuclear pore complex. Annu Rev Cell Biol 1992; 8:495-527.

74. Akey CW. The nuclear pore complex: A macromolecular transport assembly in nuclear trafficking. In: Felherr C. ed. 1992; New York Academic 370 pp.

75. Gerace L. Molecular trafficking across the nuclear pore complex. Curr Opinion Cell Biol 1992; 4:637-645.

76. Hurt EC. The nuclear pore complex. FEBS Lett 1993; 325:76-80.

77. Neumeyer DD. The nuclear pore complex and nucleocytoplasmic transport. Curr Opinion Cell Biol 1993; 5:395-407.

78. Finlay DR, Neumeyer DD, Price TM et al. Inhibition of in vitro nuclear transport by a lectin that binds to nuclear pores. J Cell Biol 1987; 104:189-200.

79. Gerace L, Ottaviano Y, Kondor-Koch C. Identification of a major polypeptide of the nuclear pore complex. J Cell Biol 1982; 95:826-837.

80. Wozniak RW, Bartnik E, Blobel G. Primary structure analysis of an integral membrane glycoprotein of the nuclear pore. J Cell Biol. 1989; 108:2083-2092.

81. Wozniak RW, Blobel G. The transmembrane segment and cyto/nucleoplasmic tail of gp210 are both necessary and sufficient for the targeting of a membrane protein to the nuclear pore. J Cell Biol 1991; 115:458a.

82. Greber UF, Gerace L. Nuclear protein import is inhibited by an antibody to a lumenal epitope of a nuclear pore complex glycoprotein. J Cell Biol. 1992; 116:15-30.

83. Pandey S, Karande AA, Mishra K et al. Inhibition of nuclear protein import by a monoclonal antibody against a novel class of nuclear pore proteins. Exp Cell Res 1994; 212:243-254.

84. D'Onofrio M, Starr CM, Park MK et al. Partial cDNA sequence encoding a nuclear pore protein modified by O-linked N-acetylglucosamine. Proc Natl Acad Sci USA 1988; 85:9595-9599.

85. Starr CM, D'Onofrio M, Park MK et al. Primary sequence and heterologous expression of nuclear pore glycoprotein. J Cell Biol 1990; 110:1861-1871.

86. Cordes V, Waizenegger I, Krohne G. Nuclear pore complex glycoprotein p62 of Xenopus laevis and mouse: cDNA cloning and identification of its glycosylated region. Eur J Cell Biol 1991; 55:31-47.

87. Sukegawa J, Blobel G. A nuclear pore complex protein that contains zinc finger motifs, binds DNA and faces the nucleoplasm. Cell 1993; 72:29-38.

88. Wente SR, Rout RP, Blobel G. A new family of yeast nuclear pore complex proteins. J Cell Biol 1992; 119:705-723.

89. Loeb JDJ, Davis LI, Fink GR. NUP2, a novel yeast nucleoporin, has functional overlap with other proteins of the nuclear pore complex. Mol Biol Cell 1993; 4:209-222.

90. Wimmer C, Doye V, Grandi P et al. A new class of nucleoporins that functionally interact with nuclear proteins NSP1. EMBO J 1992; 11:5051-5061.

91. Michalak M, Milner RE, Burns K et al. Calreticulin. Biochem J 1992; 285:681-692.

92. Sontheimer RD, Lieu T-S, Capra JD. Calreticulin the diverse functional repertoire of a new human autoantigen. The Immunologist 1993; 45:155-160.

93. Hensel G, Assman V, Kern HF. Hormonal regulation of protein disulfide isomerase and chaperone synthesis in the rat exocrine pancreas. Eur J Cell Biol 1994; 63:208-218.

94. Jethmalani SM, Henle KJ, Kaushal GP. Heat shock-induced prompt glycosylation. Identification of P-SG67 as calreticulin. J Biol Chem 1994; 269:23603-23609.

95. Jethmalani SM, Henle KJ. Prompt glycosylation of calreticulin is independent of Ca^{2+} homeostasis. Biochem Biophys Res Comm 1994; 205:780-787.

96. Plakidou-Dymock S, McGivan JD. Calreticulin-a stress protein induced in the renal epithelial cell line NBL-1 by amino acid deprivation. Cell Calcium 1994; 16:1-8.

97. Eggleton P, Lieu TS, Zappi EG et al. Calreticulin is released from activated neutrophils and binds to Clq and mannan-binding protein. Clin Immun Immun 1994; 72:405-409.

98. Zhu J, Newkirk MM. Viral induction of the human autoantigens calreticulin. Clin Invst Med 1994; 17:196-205.

99. Nakhasi HL, Singh NK, Pogue GP et al. Identification and characterization of host factor interactions with cis-acting elements of rubella virus RNA. Arch Vir 1994; 9:255-267.

100. Boehm J, Orth T, Van Nguyen P et al. Systemic lupus erythematous is associated with increased auto-antibody titers against calreticulin and grp94, but calreticulin is not the Ro/SS-A antigen. Eur J Clin Invest 1994; 24:248-257.

101. Lu J, Willis AC, Sim RB. A calreticulin-like protein co-purifies with a '60 kD' component of Ro/SS-A, but is not recognized by antibodies in Sjogren's syndrome sera. Clin Exp Immunol 1993; 94:429-434.

102. Yokoi T, Nagayama S, Kajiwara R et al. Identification of protein disulfide isomerase and calreticulin as autoimmune antigens in LEC strain of rats. Biochim Biophy Acta 1993; 1158:339-344.

103. McCauliffe DP, Sontheimer RD. Molecular characterization of the Ro/SS-A autoantigens. J Invest Derm 1993; 100:73S-79S.

104. Rokeach LA, Haselby JA, Meilof JF et al. Characterization of the autoantigen calreticulin. J Immunol 1991; 147:3031-3039.

105. Routsias JG, Tziofas AG, Sakarellos-Daitsiotis M et al. Calreticulin synthetic peptide analogues: anti-peptide antibodies in autoimmune rheumatic diseases. Clin Exp Immunol 1993; 91:437-441.

106. Rojiani, MV, Finlay BB, Gray et al. In vitro interaction of a polypeptide homologous to human Ro/SS-A antigen (calreticulin) with a highly conserved amino acid sequence in the cytoplasmic domain of integrin alpha subunits. Biochemistry 1991; 30:9859-9866.

107. Dedhar S. Novel functions for calreticulin: interaction with integrins and modulation of gene expression. TIBS 1994; 19:269-271.

108. Leung-Hagesteijn CY, Milankov K, Michalak M et al. Cell attachment to extracellular matrix substrates is inhibited upon downregulation of expression of calreticulin, an intracellular integrin alpha-subunit-binding protein. J Cell Sci 1994; 107:589-600.

109. Dupuis M, Schaerer E, Krause KH et al. The calcium binding protein calreticulin is a major constituent of lytic granules in cytolytic T lymphocytes. J Exp Med 1993; 177:1-7.

110. Burns K, Helgason CD, Bleackley RC et al. Calreticulin in T-lymphocytes. Identification of calreticulin in T-lymphocytes and demonstration that activation of T cells correlates with increased levels of calreticulin mRNA and protein. J Biol Chem 1992; 267:19039-19042.

111. Mookerjee BK, Chakrabarti R, Lee TP et al. Calcium uptake during mitogenic stimulation of human lymphocytes: characterization of intracellular calcium compartments and demonstration of the presence of immunoreactive calreticulin. Immunol Invest 1993; 22:415-429.

112. Clementi E, Martino G, Grimaldi LM et al. Intracellular Ca^{2+} stores of T lymphocytes: changes induced by in vitro and in vivo activation. Euro J Immunol 1994; 24:1365-1371.

113. Burns K, Duggan B, Atkinson EA et al. Modulation of gene expression by calreticulin binding to the glucocorticoid receptor. Nature 1994; 367:476-480.

114. Dedhar S, Rennie PS, Shago M et al. Inhibition of nuclear hormone receptor activity by calreticulin. Nature 1994; 367:480-483.

The following six figures show amino acid alignments for calreticulin from various sources. cDNAs encoding calreticulin were isolated from human (Genbank accession numbers: M32294, M84739), mouse (X14926); rabbit (J05138); rat (X79327, X53363, S56918); bovine brain (L13462); *Aplysia* (S51239); *C. elegans* (X59589); *X. laevis* (X67597, X67598); *D. melanogaster* (X64461), tick (U07708), *S. mansoni* (M93097); *S. japanicum* (M80524); barley (L27349, L27348); tobacco (X85382); *O. vulvalus* (M20565). The amino acid sequences of different calreticulins are extremely similar. Different residues are shown in lower case, grayscaled letters. KPEDWD sequence of Repeat A and putative glycosylation site are depicted in grayscale, upper case letters on pages 205 and 206. On page 207, endoplasmic reticulum localization signals are depicted in grayscale, upper case letters.

```
                            1            10           20            30          40
Human          MLLSVPLLLGLLGLAVA   EPAVYFKEQFLDGDGWTSRWIE-S-KHKS--DF-GKFVLSSGKFY
Mouse          MLLSVPLLLGLLGLAAA   DPAIYFKEQFLDGDaWTNRWVE-S-KHKS--DF-GKFVLSSGKFY
Rat            MLLSVPLLLGLLGLAAA   DPAIYFKEQFLDGDaWTNRWVE-S-KHKS--DF-GKFVLSSGKFY
Rabbit         MLLPVPLLLGLLGLAAA   EPVVYFKEQFLDGDGWTeRWIE-S-KHKS--DF-GKFVLSSGKFY
Brain-1                            DPTVYFKEQFLDGDGWTeRWIE-S-KHKP--DF-GKFVLSSGKFY
Brain-2        MCLNHFLLSIVLSIVLLFHFVFYICLHHIVTFLR  EetVFFseQFLtLD---lKyka-S-Kl-S--sI--REALSMSKV-
Xenopus-1                  LVLPLLAGLCIA   EPAVYFKEeFTDGDGWTQRWVE-S-KHKT--Dy-GKFkLSAGKFY
Xenopus-2                          DGDGWTQRWVE-S-KHKS--Dy-GKFkLSAGKFY
Aplysia        MKVVLLCALLGIAFA   DPtVYFKEeF--GDDWaeRWVE-S-KHKS--DL-GKFVLTAGKFY
Drosophila     MMWCKTVIVLLATVGF-IS   -AeVlKENF-DNENWedtWiy-S-KHpg-KEF-GKFVLTPGTFY
Tick                               G-t-sSAGKFY
C. elegans     MKSLCLLAIVAV-VS   -AeVYFKEEF-ndaSWekRWVq-S-KHKd--DF-GaFkLSAGKFf
Barley         LLRRLALLALASVAAV   aAdVfFqEKF-E-DGWeSRWVEKSWKKde-nMAGewnhTSGKWh
Tobacco                            eVFFEESFN--DGWeSRWVkSewKKde-nMAGewnHTSGKWN
S. mansoni     MLSILLTL-LLSKYAL   gheVwFsETF-pNES-ienWVq-S-tynaekq--GeFkVeAGKsp
S. japanica                        FkIeAGKSP
RAL-1          MQLSLLVGLVCFSAI   nAkIYFKEdF-sdDdWekRWIk-S-KHKd-Df--GKWeIStGKFY
```

```
                    50        60        70        80        90       100       110       120
                    -         -         -         -         -         -         -         -
Human        GDEEKDKGLQTSQDARFYALSASF-E-PFSNKGQTLVVQFTVKHEQNIDCGGGYVKLFPNSLDQTDMHGDSEYNI
Mouse        GDlEKDKGLQTSQDARFYALSAKF-E-PFSNKGQTLVVQFTVKHEQNIDCGGGYVKLFPSGLDQkDMHGDSEYNI
Rat          GDqEKDKGLQTSQDARFYALSARF-E-PFSNKGQTLVVQFTVKHEQNIDCGGGYVKLFPGGLDQkDMHGDSEYNI
Rabbit       GDqEKDKGLQTSQDARFYALSARF-E-PFSNKGQpLVVQFTVKHEQNIDCGGGYVKLFPaGLDQkDMHGDSEYNI
Brain-1      GDqEKDKGLQTSQDARFYALSARF-E-PFSNKGQTLVVQFTVKHEQNIDCGGGYVKLFPaGLDQTDMHGDSEYNI
Brain-2      GiiE-n--F-CFSEIsF-LQesI-k-sHGrRTlvgcspWG-HeEQNIDCGGGYNVFPaGLDQTDMHGDSEYNI
Xenopus-1    GDsEKDKGLQTSQDARFYAMSsRF-D-sFSNKdQTLVVQFSVKHEQNIDCGGGYVKLFPaaLEQTEMHeESEYNI
Xenopus-2    GDsEKDKGLQTSQDARFYAMSsRF-E-sFSNKdQTLVIQFSVKHEQNIDCGGGYVKLFPadLEQTEMHGESEYNI
Aplysia      GDaEKDKGIQTSQDARFYglSAkF-D-kFSNeGkTLVIQFTVKHEQNIDCGGGYVKFssDlDQSDMHGESpYNI
Drosophila   NDaEaDKGITSQDARFYAASRKF-D-gFSNedkpLVVQFSVKHEQNIDCGGGYVKLFdCSLDQTDMHGESpYeI
Tick         GDaEKsKGLQTSeDARFYgIsSKF-E-PFSNeGkTLVVQFTVKHEQNIDCGGGYVKLFdCSLDQTqMHGESpYkI
C. elegans   dvEsRDgGIQTSQDAKFYsRaAKF-D-dFSNKGkTLVIQYTVKHEQGIDCGGGYVKVMradADlGDFHGETpYNV
Barley       GDaE-DKGIQTSeDYRFYAISAey-p-eFSNKdkTlVLQFTVKHEQkLDCGGGYVKLLgGdVDQkkFgGDTpYGI
Tobacco      GDan-DKGIQTSEDYRFFAISAeF-p-eFSNKGkNLVFQFSVKHEQklDCGGGYMKLLSGdVDQKkFgGDTpYGI
S. mansoni   vDpieDlGLkTTQDARFYgIarKISE-PFSNRGkTMVLQFTVKfdkTVsCGGaYIKLLgsdIIDpkkFHGESpYkI
S. japanica  vnpieDlGLkTTQDARFYgIarKISE-PFSNRdkTLVLQFTVKfdkTVfCGGaYIKLLgsdIIDpktFHGETpYkI
RAL-1        GDavDKGLkTTQDAKFYsIGAkF-DksFSNKGkSLVIQFSVKHEQdIDCGGGYVKLMASDVnleDsHGETpyhI
```

```
                   130       140       150       160       170       180       190
                   -         -         -         -         -         -         -
Human         MFGPDICGPGTKKVHVIFNYKGKNVLINKDIRCKDDEFTHLYTLIVRPDNTYEVKIDNSQVESGSLEDDWDFLPP
Mouse         MFGPDICGPGTKKVHVIFNYKGKNVLINKDIRCKDDEFTHLYTLIVRPDNTYEVKIDNSQVESGSLEDDWDFLPP
Rat           MFGPDICGPGTKKVHVIFNYKGKNVLINKDIRCKDDEFTHLYTLIVRPDNTYEVKIDNSQVESGSLEDDWDFLPP
Rabbit        MFGPDICGPGTKKVHVIFNYKGKNVLINKDIRCKDDEFTHLYTLIVRPDNTYEVKIDNSQVESGSLEDDWDFLPP
Brain-1       MFGPDICGPGTKKVHVIFNYKGKNVLINKDIRCKDDEFTHLYTLIVRPnNTYEVKIDNSQVESGSLEDDWDFLPP
Brain-2       MFGPDICGPGTKKVHVIFNYKGKNVLINKDIRCKDDEFTHLYTLIVRPnNTYEVKIDNSQVESGSLEDDWDFLPP
Xenopus-1     MFGPDICGPpTKKVHVIFQYKKKNLqINKDIRCKDDsFTHLYTLIVRPDNTYEVKIDNSkVESGSLEDDWDFLPP
Xenopus-2     MFGPDICGPpTKKVHVIFQYKKKNLqINKDIRCKDDsFTHLYTLIVRPDNTYEVKIDNSkVESGSLEEDWDFLPP
APlysia       MFGPDICGPGTKKVHVIFNYKGKNLLVkKDIRCKDDvFSHLYTLIVRPDNTYEVKIDNekAESGDLEaDWDFLPA
Drosophila    MFGPDICGPGTKKVHVIFSYKGKNhLISKDIRCKDDvYTHFYTLIVRPDNTYEVlIDNekVESGNLEDDWDFLAP
Tick          MFPPDICGPGTKKVHVIFNYKGKNhLINKEIRCKDDvFTHLYTLIVKPDNTYvVKIDNevAEkGeLESDWSFLPP
C. elegans    MFGPDICGP-TRRVHVILNYKGeNkLIkKEItCKsDELTHLYTLILnsDNTYEVKIDGeSAqTGSLEEDWDLLPA
Barley        MFGPDICGySTKKVHtILTknGKNhLIkKDVpCetDqLSHVYTLIIRPDaTYsIlIDNeekqTGSIyEhWDILPP
Tobacco       MFGPDICGySTKKVHAILTYndtNhLIkKEVpCetDQLTHVYTFILRPDATYsIlIDNVEkqSGSLysDWDLLPP
S. mansoni    MFGPDICGmaTKKVHVIFNYKGKNhLIkKEMpCKDDlkTHLYTLIVnPnNkYEVlVDNakVEeGSLEDDWDMLPP
S. japanica   MFGPDICGmaTKRIHVIFNYKGqNhLIkKDIpCKDDqkTHLYTLIVRPDNsYEVlVDNekVESGlLEEDWnMLAP
RAL-1         MFGPDICGPGTKKVHVIFhYkdRNhMIkKDIRCKDDvFTHLYTLIVnsDNTYEVqIDGekAESGELEaDWDFLPP
```

```
         200       210       220       230       240       250       260       270

Human        KKIKDPDASKPEDWDERAKIDDPTDSKPEDWDK-PEHIPDPDAKKPEDWDEMDGEWEPPVIQNPEYKGEWKPRQ
Mouse        KKIKDPDAAKPEDWDERAKIDDPTDSKPEDWDK-PEHIPDPDAKKPEDWDEMDGEWEPPVIQNPEYKGEWKPRQ
Rat          KKIKDPDAAKPEDWDERAKIDDPTDSKPEDWDK-PEHIPDPDAKKPEDWDEMDGEWEPPVIQNPEYKGEWKPRQ
Rabbit       KKIKDPDASKPEDWDERAKIDDPTDSKPEDWDK-PEHIPDPDAKKPEDWDEMDGEWEPPVIQNPEYKGEWKPRQ
Brain-1      KKIKDPDAAKPEDWDDRAKIDDPTDSKPEDWDK-PEHIPDPDAKKPEDWDEMDGEWEPPVIQNPEYKGEWKPRQ
Brain-2      KKIKDPDAAKPEDWDDRAKIDDPTDSKPEDWDK-PEHIPDPDAKKPEDWDEMDGEWEPPLIQNPEYKGEWKPRQ
Xenopus-1    KKIKDPEAkKPEDWDERPKIDDPeDkKPEDWEK-PEHIPDPDAVKPEDWDEMDGEWEPPVIQNPEYKGEWKPRQ
Xenopus-2    KKIKDPEAkKPDDWDERPKIDDPeDkKPEDWEK-PEHIPDPDAVKPEDWDEMDGEWEPPVIQNPDlqGEWKPRQ
Aplysia      KTIPDPDAkKPDDWDEReKIDDPdDTKPEDWDK-PEHIPDPEAKKPDDWDEMDGEWEPPMIdNPEYKGEWKPKQ
Drosophila   KKIKDPtATKPEDDWDRAtIpDPdDkKPEDWDK-PEHIPDPDATKPEDWDEMDGEWEPPMIdNPEFKGEWqPKQ
Tick         KKIKDPEAkKPEDWDDRAKIDDPeDkKPEDWDK-PEyIPDPDATKPEDWDDMDGEWEPPqINNPEYKGEWKPKQ
C. elegans   KKIKDPDAkKPEDWDEReyIDDaeDaKPEDWEK-PEHIPDPDAKKPEDWDEMDGEWEPPMIdNPEYKGEWKPKQ
Barley       KeIKDPEAkKPEDWDKeyIpDPeDvKPEgyDdIPkeVtDPDAKKPEDWDEeDGEWtAPtIpNPEYKGpWKqKk
Tobacco      KTIKDPsAkKPEDWDEKEFIDDPEDKKPEgyDdIPEeItDPDAKKPEDWDqeDGEWtAPTIPNPEYKGpWKPKk
S. mansoni   KKIdDPndkKPDDWvDeQfIDDPdDkKPDnWDq-PktMPDMDAKKPDDWDaMDGEWErPqkdNPEYKGEWtPRr
S. japanica  KmIdDPndkKPDDsqEeeyIDDPNDeKPlDWDK-PktIPDMDAKKPDDWDDMDGEWkrPekhNPEYKGEWsPRr
RAL-1        KKIKDPDAkKPEDWDEReFIDDedDkKPEDWDK-PEHIPDPDAKKPEDWDDEMDGEWEPPMVdNPEYKGEWKPKQ
```

```
             280       290       300       310       320       330       340
              |         |         |         |         |         |         |
Human        IDNPDYKGTWIHPEIDNPEYSPDPSIYAYDNFGVLGLDLWQVKSGTIFDNFLITNDEAYAEEFGNETWGVTKAAE
Mouse        IDNPDYKGTWIHPEIDNPEYSPDANIYAYDSFaVLGLDLWQVKSGTIFDNFLITNDEAYAEEFGNETWGVTKAAE
RAT          IDNPDYKGTWIHPEIDNPEYSPDANIYAYDSFaVLGLDLWQVKSGTIFDNFLITNDEAYAEEFGNETWGVTKAAE
Rabbit       IDNPDYKGTWIHPEIDNPEYSPDANIYAYDSFaVLGLDLWQVKSGTIFDNFLITNDEAYAEEFGNETWGVTKTAE
Brain-1      IDNPEYKGiWIHPEIDNPEYSPDsNIYAYENFaVLGLDLWQVKSGTIFDNFLITNDEAYAEEFGNETWGVTKAAE
Brain-2      IDNPEYKGiWIHPEIDNPEYSPDsNIYAYENFaVLGLDLWQVKSGTIFDNFLITNDEAYAEEFGNETWGVTKAAE
Xenopus-1    IDNPDYKGkWIHPEIDNPEYTPDdTLYsYDSFGVLGLDLWQVKSGTIFDNFLMTNDEkhAEEyGNETWGVTKeAE
Xenopus-2    IDNPDYKGkWIHPEMDNPEYTPDsTLYsYESFGVIGLDLWQVKSGTIFDNFLMTNDEkYAEEYGNETWGVTKeAE
Aplysia      VDNPDYKGkWVHPEIDNPEYeADdKLYsfadFGAIGFDLWQVKAGTIFDNVLITdsveYAEEFGNETWGkTKdpE
Drosophila   LDNPnYKGaWeHPEIaNPEYvPDdkLYLrkeICtLGFDLWQVKSGTIFDNVLITdDveLAaKAAAEVKN-TqAgE
Tick         IDNPaYKGaWVHPEIDNPEYTADPkLYhfpeLCtIGFDLWQVKSGTIFDNLLITdDEeYArvHGeETWAALKdeE
C. elegans   IkNPaYKGkWIHPEIENPEYTPDdeLYsYESWGAIGFDLWQVKSGTIFDNIIITdsveeAEahaaETFdklKtVE
Barley       IkNPnYqGkWkaPmIaNPDfQdDPYIYAfDSLkyIGIELWQVKSGTLFDNILITdDaAlAktFaeETWAkhKdAE
Tobacco      IkNPnYKGkWkaPlIDNPDFKDDPDLYVFPNLKYVG-----Ve------IVICdDpeYAkaIAeETWGkQkdAE
S. mansoni   IDNPkYKGeWkpVqIDNPEYkhDPeLYVlndIGyVGFDLWQVdSGSIFDNILITdspdfAkEGerlW---rKryD
S. japanica  IENPkYKGQWkpAqIDNPDYkPDPeLYIQDdIGyVGFDLWQVdSGSIFDNILITdspdfAkqeGerlW---rKrhD
RAL-1        kkNPaYKGkWIHPEIEiPDYTPDdNLYVYDdIGAIGFDLWQVKSGTIFDdVIVTdsveeAkkFGekTLkITReGE
```

```
              350       360       370       380       390       400       410
               |         |         |         |         |         |         |
Human       KQMKDKQDEEQRLKEEEEDKKRKEEEAEDKEDD-EDKDEDEDEEDKEEEDEEEDVP-GQAKDEL
Mouse       KQMKDKQDEEQRLKEEEEDKKRKEEEAEDKEDD-DDRDEDEDEEDEKEEDEEE-P--GQAKDEL
Rat         KQMKDKQDEEQRLKEEEEDKKRKEEEAEDKEDD-DDRDEDEDEEDEKEED-EEDAT-GQAKDEL
Rabbit      KQMKDKQDEEQRLKEEEEKKRKEEEAEEdEEDKDDKEDEDEEDKDEEEEAA--GQAKDEL
Brain-1     KQMKDKQDEEQRLHEEEEKKgKEEEEA-DKDDD-EDKDEDEDEKEEEEEEDAAAGQAKDEL
Brain-2     KQMKDKQDEEQRLHEEEEKKgKEEEAE-KDDD-EDKDEDEDEDEKEEEEEDAAA-QAKDEL
Xenopus-1   KkMKEqQDEdRkKqEEEEKtRK-EEEpQeEDE-DDdDEEKkEEEEEEDE----TLKDEL
Xenopus-2   KkMKEqQDEEdRkKqEDEEnKqKEE-EpqEeEDD-DEeKEEE--EEEEEDE------TKDEL
Aplysia     KkMKDaQDEEdRkarEEEEKKRKEEEDAnkdDEE-EEaEEEEEEDD------AKDEL
Drosophila  KkMKEaQDEVQRkKDEEEAKKasDkQDeDEdDDD-EEKDDEskqD-------QSHDEL
Tick        KkMKEKQEEEedAKsKkEDda-KDEDEfEDeEKE-EDKEkEDEEtpEDDD------HHEL
C. elegans  KekKEKaDEEtRkaEEEarK-KaEEEkeakKDDD-EEekEEEEg-------HDEL
Barley      KaAfD---EaEkK-KEEEDasK-agEDD-DD1DDE-DadDEDkDkDEDDD------HDEL
Tobacco     KaAFE--EaEkK-REEEE-sK-aApaDsDaeEDD-DadDDADDaDDklEskD-----DEARDEL
S. mansoni  aeVakeQssakddKEEaEEtKerKElpyDaKasD-Ep--------------SGHDEL
S. japanica neLaEdQsAtksdsDkEtDKaaEEptEeDEdvkpaEnp---------------SGHDEL
RAL-1       Kk-KGKktkkQK-KkEkNEKikkEkmkkrkRanrKk
```

INDEX

Page numbers in italics denote figures (f) or tables (t).

MOLECULAR BIOLOGY
INTELLIGENCE UNIT

AVAILABLE AND UPCOMING TITLES

Neuroscience Intelligence Unit

Available and Upcoming Titles

- Neurodegenerative Diseases and Mitochondrial Metabolism
  M. Flint Beal, Harvard University

- Molecular and Cellular Mechanisms of Neostriatum
  Marjorie A. Ariano and D. James Surmeier, Chicago Medical School

- Ca²⁺ Regulation By Ca²⁺-Binding Proteins in Neurodegenerative Disorders
  Claus W. Heizmann and Katharina Braun, University of Zurich, Federal Institute for Neurobiology, Magdeburg

- Measuring Movement and Locomotion: From Invertebrates to Humans
  Klaus-Peter Ossenkopp, Martin Kavaliers and Paul Sanberg, University of Western Ontario and University of South Florida

- Triple Repeats in Inherited Neurologic Disease
  Henry Epstein, University of Texas-Houston

- Cholecystokinin and Anxiety
  Jacques Bradwejn, McGill University

- Neurofilament Structure and Function
  Gerry Shaw, University of Florida

- Molecular and Functional Biology of Neurotropic Factors
  Karoly Nikolics, Genentech

- Prion-related Encephalopathies: Molecular Mechanisms
  Gianluigi Forloni, Istituto di Ricerche Farmacologiche "Mario Negri"-Milan

- Neurotoxins and Ion Channels
  Alan Harvey, A.J. Anderson and E.G. Rowan, University of Strathclyde

- Analysis and Modeling of the Mammalian Cortex
  Malcolm P. Young, University of Oxford

- Free Radical Metabolism and Brain Dysfunction
  Irène Ceballos-Picot, Hôpital Necker-Paris

- Molecular Mechanisms of the Action of Benzodiazepines
  Adam Doble and Ian L. Martin, Rhône-Poulenc Rorer and University of Alberta

- Neurodevelopmental Hypothesis of Schizophrenia
  John L. Waddington and Peter Buckley, Royal College of Surgeons-Ireland

- Synaptic Plasticity in the Retina
  H.J. Wagner, Mustafa Djamgoz and Reto Weiler, University of Tübingen

- Non-classical Properties of Acetylcholine
  Margaret Appleyard, Royal Free Hospital-London

- Molecular Mechanisms of Segmental Patterning in the Vertebrate Nervous System
  David G. Wilkinson, National Institute of Medical Research-UK

- Molecular Character of Memory in the Prefrontal Cortex
  Fraser Wilson, Yale University

MEDICAL INTELLIGENCE UNIT

AVAILABLE AND UPCOMING TITLES

DATE DUE

DEMCO, INC. 38-2971